Samuel Lee Oliver, MDiv, BCC

What the Dying Teach Us
Lessons on Living

*Pre-publication
REVIEWS,
COMMENTARIES,
EVALUATIONS . . .*

"**T**heory can teach us some things, but experience is an indispensable teacher in all things, especially in ministry to the dying. Learn from the experience of Sam Lee Oliver, whose dedication to his ministry as a hospice pastoral counselor is evident in every line of *What the Dying Teach Us.* Pastor Oliver teaches his readers how to learn from the dying, for they are a font of wisdom in an age that wants to know how to help people die with dignity and peace.

He has discovered from his experience that the dying are partners in this ministry. Learn from Pastor Oliver and his patients what it means to journey to a peaceful and dignified death."

Keith J. Egan, PhD
*J. M. Hank Aquinas Professor
in Catholic Theology,
St. Mary's College;
Adjunct Professor in Theology,
Notre Dame University,
Notre Dame, IN*

More pre-publication
REVIEWS, COMMENTARIES, EVALUATIONS . . .

"**S**am Oliver has been gifted with a listening heart and has gained important insights from his patients. He shares these insights in a way that is both accessible and moving. Each brief chapter focuses on a particular lesson and can easily be used as a meditation for one's self or with others."

Laurel Arthur Burton, ThD
Professor of Religion and Medicine,
Rush-Presbyterian-St. Luke's
Medical Center,
Chicago, Il.

"**S**am Oliver's book, *What the Dying Teach Us: Lessons on Living,* is seemingly a book about death, but actually it is about life. Some books come from the mind of the author; Sam's book comes from his heart. I felt as though I was given a special invitation to be with Sam and his hospice family and friends as they ventured into the depth of life and probed its secrets. What a rare opportunity to allow myself to be taught by those who faced the great unknown. Sam Oliver is a loving and compassionate companion not only for those he serves, but for those who read *What the Dying Teach Us: Lessons on Living.*"

Jim Rosemergy
Unity Minister,
Executive Vice President,
Unity School of Christianity,
Unity Village, MO

"**O**liver's attentiveness to real people who are dying has given us an important bridge between their lives and ours. We can no longer be comfortable with dividing the world into the two camps of 'us' and 'them,' but are forced to see 'us' *in* 'them.' Their experiences with the process of dying can help us with the process of living, if we will listen. This is a real-life look at real-life people, seen through a pastoral lens."

Benjamin P. Bogia, MDiv, PhD
Associate Professor and Director,
Division of Clinical Pastoral Counseling,
University of Kentucky,
Lexington, KY

"**O**liver gives very significant insights into the spiritual pathways that all of us express and experience. . . . He offers patient care, definitions, inspiration, and hope that we might embrace our mortality, or the dying of someone we love or someone in our care. This book will be a friend to patients and families and a helpful guide to professionals and volunteers to provide much-needed support."

Rev. Fr. Richard P. Gilbert
Executive Director,
Connections-Spiritual Links,
Valparaiso, IN

The Haworth Pastoral Press
An Imprint of The Haworth Press, Inc.

What the Dying Teach Us
Lessons on Living

THE HAWORTH PASTORAL PRESS
Religion and Mental Health
Harold G. Koenig, MD
Senior Editor

New, Recent, and Forthcoming Titles:

A Gospel for the Mature Years: Finding Fulfillment by Knowing and Using Your Gifts by Harold Koenig, Tracy Lamar, and Betty Lamar

Is Religion Good for Your Health? The Effects of Religion on Physical and Mental Health by Harold Koenig

Adventures in Senior Living: Learning How to Make Retirement Meaningful and Enjoyable by J. Lawrence Driskill

Dying, Grieving, Faith, and Family: A Pastoral Care Approach by George W. Bowman

The Pastoral Care of Depression: A Guidebook by Binford W. Gilbert

Understanding Clergy Misconduct in Religious Systems: Scapegoating, Family Secrets, and the Abuse of Power by Candace R. Benyei

What the Dying Teach Us: Lessons on Living by Samuel Lee Oliver

What the Dying Teach Us
Lessons on Living

Samuel Lee Oliver, MDiv, BCC

The Haworth Pastoral Press
An Imprint of The Haworth Press, Inc.
New York • London

The Haworth Press, Inc., 10 Alice Street, Binghamton, NY 13904-1580

Cover design by Monica L. Seifert.

"Painting Pictures We Cannot See," "Lessons of Hope from the Dying," "I'll Be with You," "Healing Moments," "Where the Soul Never Dies," "Eternal Love," "A Transformed Life," "Words of God," "The Freeing Power of Questions," "Lamaze Lessons for the Soul," "Keeping the Magic Alive," "Creating Spiritual Awareness," "Spiritual Ethics in the Medical Setting," "Soul Retrieval," and "Perceptions of Reality and Death" are reprinted by permission of Prime National Publishing Corporation. Copyright © 1994, 1995, 1996, 1997.

Library of Congress Cataloging-in-Publication Data

Oliver, Samuel Lee.
   What the dying teach us : lessons on living / Samuel Lee Oliver.
      p. cm.
   Includes bibliographical references and index.
   ISBN 0-7890-0476-3 (alk. paper)
   1. Terminally ill—Pastoral counseling of. 2. Terminally ill—Religious life. 3. Death—Religious aspects—Christianity. I. Title.
BV4338.O57 1998
259'.4—dc21   97-43515
                                                        CIP

I dedicate this book, and the poems within it, to the many hospice patients and their families who have shared with me so many spiritual events and valuable lessons, and to my family: Holly, Emilee, and Luke Oliver.

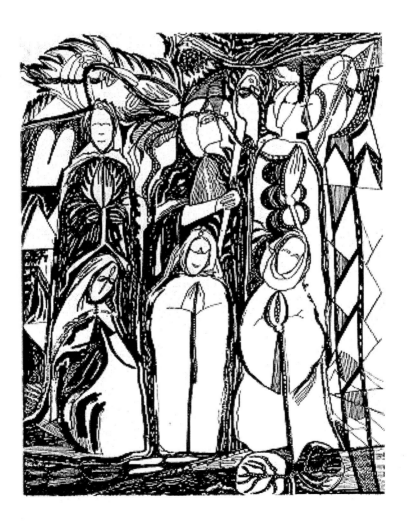

ABOUT THE AUTHOR

Reverend Samuel Lee Oliver, BCC, is a Pastoral Counselor at the Hospice of St. Joseph County, Inc. in South Bend, Indiana, and Chair of the Hospice Ethics Committee. He also serves as the State Continuing Education Chair for the College of Chaplains. Reverend Oliver is a member and contributing writer with the *Editorial Review Board for Healing Ministry Journal* and a board member of the *American Journal of Hospice and Palliative Care.* He has written numerous articles that have appeared in *Enlightenments, Healing Ministry Journal, Explorer Magazine,* and in various poetry anthologies. Reverend Oliver began teaching and speaking about providing spiritual care to the dying five years ago and continues to speak at public engagements on the national and international levels.

CONTENTS

Foreword

Several years ago, I delivered an unpublished paper to a group of churches in northwest Indiana. The paper was intended to help them understand why they were being asked to contribute large sums of money to our denomination's new church in the center of our association of churches. The new church was young: over 50 percent of its members were eighteen years of age or less. And, as one might imagine, given the age of its membership, this church was poor—very poor. Beyond that, it was a multiracial (predominantly African-American) church in a mostly white, midwestern small town. They had little capital, and most of its members were transplants from a nearby metropolitan area. The church's ministry did not contain a strong church-growth component and the primary focus was on the marginalized, the poor, the homeless, and those incarcerated in the county jail or in a neighboring state prison. The pastor let it be known to the community's funeral directors that he would be glad to do memorial services for the derelicts who could not afford a traditional funeral. Demographically, and in almost every other way, this church should have failed, for according to all the principles of church growth, this fledgling congregation had everything against it and did almost everything wrong.

I wrote the paper to gain broad-based spiritual and financial support for the new church. I figured those of us in the long-established and more affluent congregations would be able to provide moral and monetary support for them. Little did I know how much they would teach us about being the Church. I thought they needed me and others like me to support their efforts lest their efforts go unnoticed or be ineffective. I soon learned that they were not going to become the "project" of a group of do-gooder congregations. But most important, I discovered that I needed to listen to them and take them seriously.

This congregation taught me at least two things. First, it taught me that the world's definition of a faith community and faith's definition of a faith community can be very different. The faith communities to which many of us belong, by and large, are shaped by our culture. The expectations we have about ministries, norms, and mores are shaped by the world around us and woven into the very fabric of our lives. On the other hand, the church, synagogue, or mosque that takes its faith seriously refuses to become like the culture around it. It becomes an alternative community. This was precisely what this congregation became, a faithful alternative to the religious expressions that smacked more of this world than of faith.

Second, these people taught me that the words in Christian scripture (the Lord said to me) ". . . 'my power is made perfect in weakness' . . . For the sake of Christ, then, I am content with weaknesses, insults, hardships, persecutions, and calamities; for when I am weak, then I am strong" (2 Corinthians 12:9-10) are true. I had become trapped in some old patterns of thinking, thinking that was more attuned to what the world deems an appropriate definition of strength and weakness. I had forgotten that if you really want to learn about strength, you may want to check in with those who are weak. If you want to know what it means to be whole, you may want to check in with those who are broken. And in that time together, you would do well to listen, to yield to what you see, hear, and feel. And, if you can, embrace it for awhile and allow it to have its way with you. You will be amazed at how much you will learn about living from those who are weak, broken, and dying.

In Sam Oliver's book, *What the Dying Teach Us,* we are invited to enter two worlds—both of which are broken, both of which experience the grace of healing love. The first is the lives of those dying persons with whom pastoral counselor Sam Oliver spent much time and energy in ministry. We are asked to sit with, and, in a sense, dialogue with persons such as Iris, Skeet, Bob, and their families and friends as they wrestle with a primary spiritual issue—how can I/we find life and meaning in the face of death. If we are open to these stories of courage and grace we will learn alot. Our lives may even be changed.

But we are also encouraged to enter the author's world, to see his soul. Unabashedly, Sam allows us in to hear his misgivings, his doubts, the questions he raises with himself and God about living and dying.

Those who have been spiritual caregivers will readily identify with Sam. We have been there, and he helps us see again what we know already from our experience but refuse to believe, that somehow God's power is made perfect in weakness—our congregants' weakness and our own. Those who have been primary caregivers for dying persons will be warmed and strengthened to know that they are not alone in their weakness: their feelings of inadequacy, their fears, their perplexities, their sense of failure, the almost daily roller-coaster ride of the best and the worst experiences and feelings that humanity can have. For those who are facing their death in the imminent future, who live daily with chemotherapy, radiation, hair loss, nausea, bandanas, anger, confusion, scores of persons who do not understand, and everything else that may accompany their final months or weeks of life, they will learn to yield themselves up to the holy; to release the grasp they have had for so long on the things of this world, as if this world could save them, and to find that in the very thing that is killing them, there will be strength!

This book will speak to many, and it may even provide some answers. But they will not be answers of this world, for the world does not abide weakness, brokenness, and death. Those whom we meet in this book help us realize that the ultimate answers about life are found not in all the "stuff" of life we hold onto tenaciously. The ultimate answers of life are discerned best in a journey characterized by, of all things, brokenness.

Reverend Doctor Alva F. Hohl Jr.
Pastor, Zion United Church of Christ
South Bend, Indiana

Acknowledgments

I wish to thank my wife, friends, and co-workers who spent many hours listening to me talk about this book. A special thank you to Holly Oliver, Mark Murray, Roberta Spencer, Steve Nani, and Kate Lee for reading each story and commenting on them. My life has been touched by these who patiently encouraged me. I offer a special thanks to my friend, Susan, for her gift. I am grateful to April Ford and Cheryl Szucsits for their excellent artwork. And, I want to thank the patients and families who have given me these stories to share. Without them, I would not have been so inspired to complete this writing. Most important, I wish to thank God, whose Spirit has guided me through the completion of this project.

I have been blessed, and my life has been changed as a result. I learned that the success of this project and any other project is not determined by its popularity or unpopularity. Rather, its prosperity is determined by the knowledge and wisdom I have gained, plus the lessons I have learned about living through the experiences of others. In this regard, I thank each person who has taught me how to live.

Introduction

In this book, you will find mystery, joy, and sorrow. It contains journeys of real people—hospice patients and their families—whom I've met as a pastoral care counselor.

What the Dying Teach Us is a collection of actual experiences and insights from the terminally ill. We have a great deal to learn from the dying about hope, values, and faith. Their experiences teach us valuable lessons about giving and affirming life. The stories I have selected are more than intellectual conceptions of life. These stories will touch your heart and renew your soul. They are . . .

"Healing Words"

Words draw out concepts
which articulate perceptions
of a person, place, or thing.

Each give rise to meaning
and describe a particular aspect
of the relationship that has surfaced.

To transcend ordinary vocalizations
is to recognize the sentient nature
revealed in life's rhythm.

These vibrations lead the heart
into areas of the soul
where connections are eternal.

Sam Oliver

PART ONE:
LESSONS ON HEALING,
HOPE, AND PEACE

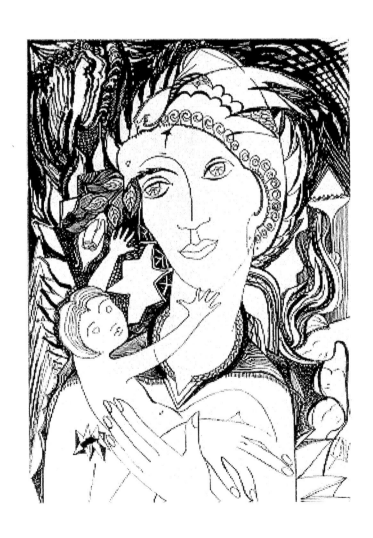

A Moment of Grace

Lesson 1: The difference between one who experiences grace and one who does not is a shift in conscious awareness.

My life has provided me with many grace-filled moments. On one occasion, I was given the opportunity to visit a fifty-nine-year-old woman who was a patient with hospice. She had children and a husband whom she dearly loved. Two years prior to our meeting, she had an uncommon near-death experience that had frightened her because of her misconceptions about near-death encounters. As a hospice patient, she was aware that she would be facing death again, so she asked me to come and visit.

The first time we met she told me about her near-death experience, that had been confirmed by her physician. She told me she experienced being pulled or drawn forward through a long, dark hallway. At the end of the hallway was a door. Though something inside her felt that if she went through this door she would enter Eternity, still she fought it. Then, she found herself becoming conscious of her hospital bed.

This woman was fearful because she felt she needed to see a great light and didn't. From her readings on near-death experiences, she understood how others saw such a light. She was wondering if something was wrong, and she was fearful of what might have happened if she had entered the door at that time in her life. I tried to encourage her to simply appreciate her experience without judgment or comparison to the experiences of others. Her experience was hers and no one else's, and no one could diminish or take away her spiritual encounter. Each of us has a personal experience with God that is unlike anyone else's. This is our uniqueness. When she was finally able to appreciate her near-death experience as her own, she found freedom in that holy moment to emerse herself into depths of reality where only the spirit can travel. I thanked this hospice patient for sharing with me her moment in Eternity. I felt blessed to recall that sacred moment with her. We were on the edge of the "Mystery," and it was her spirit, recollecting in the present that took me there. We then shared a prayer to bless the moment she was able to transcend and discover a depth of reality often ignored in this life.

Many tears surfaced during our discussion. This lady did share with me that her life was never the same after that near-death event. She was forever changed. Who knows why this woman didn't die during her near-death experience. She may not have been ready, or it could be that I needed to meet her before she left this world. I might have needed to learn something from this woman I would not have learned in any other way.

About three days later, one of the hospice nurses visited her. She told her that she felt much better about her near-death experience. Although I couldn't determine anything factually, when I left her home, I had wondered if she had been experiencing a transformation process of some kind through her tears. All I can tell you is I know *I* was transformed. I have become a better pastoral care counselor for hospice within these experiences of the Sacred that mere words cannot describe.

Often the difference between one who experiences grace and one who does not is a shift in conscious awareness. Many times, I have run into trouble with events in my life where I would try to evaluate my situation instead of letting the situation simply be my experience.

About three years ago, my wife and I moved from Kentucky to northern Indiana. From the outset I believed the move was a mistake, even though I felt deeply directed in my move. I have always been one who draws much energy from nature, and Kentucky is a beautiful state. For a long while, I began to compare the landscape in these two areas of the country. It wasn't until I began to appreciate the beauty of the landscape in northern Indiana and the uniqueness it provides that I was released from clinging to my past and was able to keep my consciousness in the present moment.

Also, I tried to compare people in northern Indiana to those in Kentucky. I found I could not do this without feeling the loss or grief of not giving value to the relationships I now have in this period of my life. I am convinced that anything we do in life needs to be done to the fullest in the present moment. We need to experience everything and everyone without judgment or comparison. We need to allow each experience we have to lead us into dimensions of reality that teach us to appreciate the present and all that it contains.

PERSONAL REFLECTIONS

Healing Moments

Lesson 2: To make a spiritual connection in a situation that requires the best of who we are demands a respect for the personal relationship each person has with God apart from a dogmatic approach to ministry.

When I was a resident hospital chaplain in central Kentucky, I was asked to visit a patient on a cancer unit who doctors suspected only had hours to live. Earlier that day, the patient's wife was asked to notify the family of her husband's approaching death. Her family doctor thought it might be helpful if she wasn't alone the rest of the day.

The attending nurse had asked me to come and visit with the family and offer support and, possibly, prayer. The nurse had told me that death was close and the family was asking for a minister. I received this call from the opposite end of the hospital. It was a long walk, so I had time to anticipate and contemplate the time ahead of me.

The patient had a large family—approximately fifteen people— from the mountains of eastern Kentucky. They were in and out of the room the whole time I was present. Most of the family depended on the patient to financially support them. I remember the patient's room being very dark, and I can still see the abundance of tears that filled it as the family gathered around the patient's bed. The patient was not verbally responsive at the time of my visit.

In the midst of great sorrow, I offered a word of prayer. I only vaguely remember the exact prayer that I voiced, but I do remember praying for God's strength and guidance to be with the family in their time of need. Also, I remember the prayer being a very difficult one for me to pray. Inwardly, I felt a weight that was almost too hard for me to bear. This heaviness of heart secretly drew me to pray for this man's recovery, especially since the family needed him. I was puzzled by the conflict that was going on inside me. I felt as if it was going against the natural process of human life to ask for his recovery, since he was so close to death.

After spending some time with the family, I went back to my office to leave for home for the weekend. I didn't dwell upon this experience much during those two days, but on Monday, when I returned to work, I was quickly reminded of my time with the family. The weekend social worker, a fellow minister, had a message from the family of the patient. As it turned out, the patient wanted to thank me for the prayer I prayed on his behalf. I learned that the following Sunday, just two days after our time together, the patient had been released from the hospital. The moment I heard this, I was silent and perplexed. I was left to ponder which prayer the patient heard: my verbal prayer or the prayer I silently prayed.

I have come to believe that my inner struggle with this family's situation had a great deal to do with my lack of faith that God would provide for them in the man's absence. I may have been connecting with this family through their similar prayers for this man's restoration of life, but I will probably never know this for certain, especially since I never saw or heard from them again. One thing I am certain of is that the family made a profound impression on me. I have come to realize the need to be aware of my internal thoughts when I am with a dying patient. Did this patient hear those internal thoughts? I don't know, nor will I claim to know. Yet I do believe, when concerning matters of the soul, anything is possible.

Often, a chaplain is called to be with a family who knows little or nothing about the minister. Together, we are spontaneously emersed into a holy moment causing the chaplain to draw from every resource within him or herself. To make a connection in a situation that requires the best of who we are demands a respect for the personal relationship each person has with God apart from a dogmatic approach to ministry.

Because a chaplain does not generally have the privilege of being in a relationship with people for any length of time, it is vital for the chaplain to trust intuition for guidance. Many times, I have wondered what my prayer for this patient and his family would have been if I had known then what I know now. Nevertheless, I do carry inside me the knowledge of the important role the inner voice can play in a minister's visit. Ever since that visit with this dying man, my faith journey has been deepened by this mystery.

This particular patient taught me that beyond my counseling skills as a minister, eloquent words of prayer and compassionate demeanor is a connection with a fellow soul that transcends ordinary words to an inner dialogue. Some have called our inner selves the "divine child" or "our greater self." We talk to our inner self every day. Through self-talk, I wonder if we can use our conversations with our inner self to connect to others. I believe the connection could be another way of enhancing communication. If you and I were to utilize this particular aspect of ourselves for the spiritual comfort of others, we may unearth a language of the soul that transcends the spoken word. Certainly, within every dialogue is another conversation that takes place, but we do not share this aspect of ourselves very often. Someday after humanity is finished discovering the human potential of the mind and body and after we have maximized technological capabilities, perhaps we will be ready to flourish in the infinite eventuality of the soul.

Not long ago, I was speaking to a friend who was longing to be loved for being himself. He has AIDS, and his mother was trying to keep him from going public with the rest of the family. Meanwhile, he was in turmoil. In attempting to keep the reality of his situation at bay, the process shielded his inner self to the point that the message he received from his mother and the message he chose to tell himself isolated the very part of him that he wanted heard the most.

My friend's case mirrored the inner turmoil I felt regarding the patient I saw in Kentucky. I found great risk in sharing my inner self because I was breaking through the known areas of my life to the mystical moments that lead me to a deeper spirituality. Perhaps, when you and I can learn to define who we are from this place so deep within our being, nothing in this external world can keep us from sharing words of comfort which touch the soul.

The action of a small child might remind us of this kind of communication skill that goes beyond words. I can remember a time recently when I was sick, and lying on the couch in our living room. I felt miserable and lifeless with the flu. My rest was interrupted when I felt a cold object gently touch my nose. As I opened my eyes, I saw my twenty-one-month-old daughter, Emilee, handing me her Ernie toy that played the tune "Rock-a-Bye-Baby." Her mother and I occasionally sing this song to calm her, either at bedtime or when she needs comforting. My wife, Holly, and I have seen her try to sing this song to her favorite doll as well. I cannot tell you what was going on inside my little girl when she gave me the toy, but I can tell you that without a single word spoken, my daughter spoke volumes to my inner self. An amazing thing happened after all this—I began to feel a little better.

Did my daughter draw my conscious awareness from the effects of the flu to a place within that silently witnessed all events happening in that moment? This moment between my awareness of the flu and my daughter's actions appeared to have shifted my attention into this silent witness in my life. Once it emerged, a transforming connection to a source of life, greater than my daughter and I, seemed to have joined us in a very special way. It was a healing experience I shall never forget.

Healing moments connect us to this place so deep within our being that we are drawn by the Spirit, from the utter depths of our soul, to a dimension of existence that has neither a foundation or any such physical faculties to rest our existence. It is a presence of love lifting us to heights beyond all thought and reason, until we yield our whole self in a solitude of silence that is joined by the power of peace.

PERSONAL REFLECTIONS

I'll Be with You

LESSON 3: When the body yields itself to the soul, there is a oneness with the universe, freeing us from our dependence on the existence of this life to define us.

Now the eleven disciples went to Galilee, to the mountain to which Jesus had directed them. And when they saw him they worshiped him; but some doubted. And Jesus came and said to them, "All authority in heaven and on earth has been given to me. Go therefore and make disciples of all nations, baptizing them in the name of the Father and of the Son and of the Holy Spirit, teaching them to observe all that I have commanded you; and lo, I am with you always, to the close of the age." (Matthew 28:16-20 RSV)

In the fall of 1992, I was running in a road race just outside of Lexington, Kentucky. During the race, I reached back to rest my arms on my hips. When I did this, I felt a knot on my back. At that time I didn't think the knot was anything more than a strained muscle.

A few weeks passed and the knot was still there. Weeks turned into months, and I kept hoping the knot would simply go away. At the time, I was a resident chaplain in a cancer unit in Kentucky, and I was painfully aware of the possibility that this could be more than a pulled muscle.

A year and a half later, after moving to South Bend, Indiana, I finally decided to go see a doctor. My doctor thought it was no more than a fatty tumor, but he wasn't 100 percent sure. Also, the tumor was so close to my spine that he felt it was best to have it taken out whether it was cancerous or not.

The following week, I went into outpatient surgery to have the knot removed. Then, I had to wait about a week and a half for the test results. The wait was slow. I imagined the worst. I began worrying about future pain, being dependent on my wife to care for me, anticipating loss of future possibilities in this life, and wondering who I could talk to about my ultimate concerns for my soul. I planned my funeral among other things. These voices of worry were very loud. I think they were the loudest for me on the day I returned to the hospital for the results of the biopsy.

I was asked to sit in the waiting room until my doctor was able to see me. All of those voices from the past week surfaced and I was flooded with emotions such as fear, anger, and anticipated sorrow. I felt as if I was going to explode. Suddenly, it occurred to me that my fear was taking over my life. At that point, I decided to focus on the very basic element of life—breathing. As I followed my breathing into the center of who I am, I was led into a holy place of peace beyond my mind and emotions. In this place within, I was able to hear similar words I often tell hospice patients to listen for as they voice their fears of dying: "I'll be with you."

I was amazed at the transformation that took place within my soul when I heard the voice of God in the midst of my fears. At that moment, I began to laugh. Somehow, I forgot to listen to God's words of grace for myself that I so often share with the patients I serve. Perhaps, it is easier to offer grace than it is to receive grace. Also, God's voice can be hard to hear when we choose to give exclusive attention to the voices of fear. I can't tell you what happened inside my soul during that time, but I can tell you from that moment on I was at peace. I knew with confidence that no matter what the doctor had to say to me in his office, I knew I would be given hope beyond my present circumstances. I knew this hope would move beyond my physical domain and I would find meaning in a world without end. In this state of being, I was ready to face any challenge the world could offer. I was relieved, however, when the doctor told me the tumor was not malignant.

Others do not hear these coveted words from their doctors. Numerous people go on to hear many words from nurses, doctors, social workers, etc., about their future cancer treatments. Patients and their families hear many voices in the medical unit who try to assure them that the staff is there to care for them. Because of the various voices in the medical profession who tell the patients to trust in the healthcare system, I find the need for a chaplain's voice to be equally vital to help the patients' spirituality. The chaplain can help patients and families hear the words I heard that day in the doctor's waiting room: "I'll be with you."

Often cancer patients are told that they can no longer be as productive as they used to be due to the needed chemotherapy to help them survive. For many, this news can shatter all they have ever known life to be. If there is a redeeming factor in living with cancer, it calls on people to search for meaning and trust in a life beyond biological functioning. When the body yields itself to the soul, there is a oneness with the universe, freeing us from our dependence on the existence of this life to define us.

Not long ago, I was giving a lecture to a group of ministers on ministry to the dying. As a part of our time together, I asked them to think of three roles in their life that were most important to them, such as: minister, father, mother, etc. Then, I asked them to describe life without these roles. It didn't take long before a minister spoke up and said, "What's left?" This minister manifested exactly what I hoped would be revealed in this exercise. Finding meaning beyond our physical abilities could very well be the beginning point of ministry and holistic health care to the dying.

We live in a world where what we "do" becomes more vital than "who we are." I encounter many people who struggle to find meaning in their dying. I grieve with them as they lose the ability to function as they once did, but I am deeply saddened if they no longer find themselves valuable based on their inability to "do" certain tasks.

Frequently, the dying are embarrassed by their need to be visited by people from their church or even their minister. The dying patient doesn't want to "bother" people who are very busy. This could have some validity, but it could also be an attempt to turn away from God's grace through those who come in God's name. I try to tell the patients I visit that they have been a blessing to me. For example, I visited a man who used humor to cope with his dying. At the end of his life, he began to say his goodbyes. On one occasion, he told me that he would put a good word in to God for me when he reached heaven. He was a wonderful example of how humor can help people deal with their dying. Also, in the dying patients' encouragement of my ministry to them, I grow in my ability to minister. Therefore, I see in my visits to dying patients the opportunity to share a journey into the soul and discover with them the core of who they are. I also see an opportunity to share a journey into the presence of God, who continues to lead dying patients into a deeper dimension of their existence, to hear God's voice say, "I'll be with you."

PERSONAL REFLECTIONS

Lessons of Hope from the Dying

LESSON 4: Peace is found when people come to the end of all they know and are willing to reach out for someone or something they trust to lead them into a new and deeper realization of existence.

The room was filled with many pictures of friends and family as well as other memorabilia. It was a room where many long hours of carpentry work had taken place to create a rustic atmosphere appropriate to Henry's personality. Approaching his seventy-fifth birthday, Henry was not able to get around as he had in his early years, because of lung cancer. During Henry's last days, as he lay confined to this bedroom, he told one story after another.

Henry and I spoke often. He wasn't a very big man, but he did have a big heart. When his blue eyes looked into mine, my heart could sense his desire to connect with me in an intimate way. He was loved by his family, and I came to love him as well.

Henry had many fears about dying, and he faced those fears with great courage. Gradually, he let go of the earthly possibilities that deteriorated around him each day. He was able to look inside himself. This inner journey helped him to see more of existence than what can be observed through outward eyes. Here, Henry found hope and a world without end. For Henry, the gift of time that prolonged dying gives was a blessing. He was able to find peace in his prolonged life and move forward to the one to come.

Before Henry could take this inner journey, life as he knew it had to come to a close. In his dying, Henry never accepted letting go of this life, yet he was able to realize that death was a part of life. In fact, he taught me that acceptance isn't necessary in order to die peacefully. Honesty and integrity about how we relate to God, self, and others are important lessons to a peaceful death.

We hear a lot about accepting death as a reality. Yet, we live in a society that spends a great deal of money and time to deny death. Cartoons portray characters who fall off cliffs time after time and somehow come back to life. Some religious denominations say, "If you believe hard enough, God will heal you." There are products that will keep us looking young in a vain attempt to deny the obvious. It's time to look at death and dying in a realistic and hopeful way that does not compromise one's integrity.

To be honest or realistic about one's death does not mean that the dying process is all doom and gloom. Some have used the opportunity to reflect on their past, evaluate the present, and anticipate the future. Others have used the opportunity to mend certain relationships that have caused pain. Many dying people find that they make the most of each day. They may notice things they never have before, appreciate things or people they haven't in the past, and they may even love life for the first time. Overall, the ability to be grateful for what a person still has in the midst of loss can provide a positive outlook for the dying.

I'll never forget what a teenage boy dying of leukemia told me at a University Medical Center in central Kentucky. We were talking about insensitive comments that people make to the dying. One of his high school buddies asked him how long he had to live, and his response was, "I have until I die."

I laughed with him about that comment, but I couldn't help wondering how our own comments about others' dying reflect a personal need to acknowledge this reality in ourselves. This teenage boy's statement has affected my life to this day. His answer is my answer and your answer. How much time do we have? None of us know for sure, but we do know that we have the present. Dying people teach us that all any of us have is the present. When you and I are not fully present or honest at any given moment, we may find ourselves distant to those we love.

Another lesson of hope from the dying lies in one's integrity. *Webster's Dictionary* defines integrity as "a being complete, wholeness, soundness, etc. . . . " If we go by this definition, we need to be willing to acknowledge the whole existence of a person's life and not just part of it.

People who are dying don't have time to play games, and they know when we are not being straightforward with them. Most of the people I have met with during their dying process have seemed to appreciate it when I acknowledged their perceived good and bad points. I have found that the need to have the whole self acknowledged is important. In a sense, it is like knowing someone's true self. All of us have qualities about ourselves that could be improved upon, and many people are afraid of sharing such intimate details for fear that a part of their "self" will be rejected. It is so important to understand that when a person tells us such intimate perceptions of themselves, he or she is engaged in finding a way to express and validate their inner self. People generally want someone who will listen with a nonjudgmental ear and not try to get them to reject a part of themselves that is perceived as bad, by way of passing it off nonchalantly.

Finally, some people who are dying begin the process of looking inward for a journey that has no end. For others, this life journey does have an end. It is necessary for those who deal with the dying to listen and be taught by the dying patient as to how this part of their life will be lived out. Sometimes, it is tempting to enforce our own beliefs and values upon the dying patient, but it is important to remember that our values are our own and no matter how hard we try we cannot manipulate the inner soul of another unless he or she allows us in.

Some people find hope in knowing that pain and suffering will finally be over. For others, peace is found when they come to the end of all they know and are willing to reach out for someone or something they trust to lead them into a new and deeper realization of existence.

PERSONAL REFLECTIONS

A Transformed Life

Lesson 5: Between actuality and potentiality lies an evolutionary experience where the soul transcends space and time and enters human consciousness from the depths of infinity.

When I was in my early teens, my grandmother, Rosie Lee Sowell Johnson, taught me how to stick my finger in a biscuit and pour honey in the hole. Then, we would savor the sweet taste of honey and biscuit. The moment was ecstasy. Little did I know that some sixteen years later I would be co-officiating her funeral with my dad.

Before the funeral, I tried to formulate thoughts to describe my grandmother. Many memories of her flashed through my mind. Even though she had lived for eighty-nine years, I found the process of deciding what words to say on my grandmother's behalf rather difficult. As a pastoral care counselor for hospice, I am often asked to give eulogies on behalf of people who have died. I never imagined on the day my grandmother and I broke bread and shared a communion-like experience that I would be presenting a brief homily at her funeral. The experience will forever be in my memory.

Helping officiate at my grandmother's funeral was not as hard as I had imagined. In fact, I found myself being in a rather peculiar place spiritually. On the one hand, I felt a deep sigh of sorrow for my grandmother's life that had come to a close. Or did it? Another part of me was extremely comforted. Although my grandmother's physical life had come to an end, her spirit or the essential nature of who she really was, is, and shall ever be drew a great number of people from the community she lived.

There were many family members at grandmother's funeral who I had not seen in years. Being with them and trying to catch up on a gap of time was very energizing and renewing for me.

My joy in the midst of my sorrow drew me to a place of peace. How could I not speak of hope on that day? I could see before me a gathering of people whose lives had been transformed in some way or another. The cousins I used to play with in my grandmother's yard were now adults with children of their own. As well as my aunts and uncles, my grandfather, who was married to my grandmother some seventy years, were all in the midst of a transformation.

Each moment of our lives, we are engaged in a process of aging and growth that leads us into new dimensions of reality. From the moment you began reading this story until now, a variety of words have entered your mind formulating images and possibly evoking feelings. Even as I write these words, I am sharing with you a portion of my grandmother's life that has now become a part of your own life experience through this written word. In a sense, your life has just been transformed.

It was my grandmother's death that drew my conscious awareness to this reality. The presence of her spirit that drew everyone to her funeral led us into a place where we could join one another in recognizing that her life did have value, meaning, and purpose. At an even deeper level, my grandmother drew every one of us into the dimension of our souls that could not find peace until we rested our trust in the very wisdom that not only created my grandmother's life, but the very lives of each one of us.

In the realm of the spirit, I cannot say that my grandmother died. Sure, I have my moments of sorrow, but I do not grieve so deeply that the spirit of life doesn't come to me and comfort my soul with wisdom. I am not talking about the kind of wisdom that we acquire in this life. Rather, I am talking about the kind of wisdom revealed in eternity.

Two months after grandmother's funeral, I was in the midst of a meditation with soft music in the background. In a state of prayer, I closed my eyes and waited in silence. I was not asking for anything or praying for anything in particular. I was simply resting in silence. From the darkness within myself, a flicker of light appeared out of nowhere. At first, the flicker of light was subtle and a great distance away. As the light drew near, an image began to take shape. Suddenly, I found myself looking face to face with my grandmother. Cold chills ran through my body. Even as I remember this experience, I know I am in the midst of a holy moment of recollection.

My grandmother did not die. She was transformed into another dimension of existence. I cannot prove that any of this ever happened and I wouldn't want to even if I could. The mere fact that someone who reads this will agree that another realm of life exists beyond the physical, or that others will contemplate such an event to disprove faith in the spirit life of fellow souls, is enough.

To me, the journey of faith in the spirit life and the doubting of the possibility, both lead us to the same place. Both paths draw our attention to an awareness of thought beyond the five senses, the ego, and present perceptions of our existence. Between actuality and potentiality lies an evolutionary experience where the soul transcends space and time and enters human consciousness from the depths of infinity.

PERSONAL REFLECTIONS

Where the Soul Never Dies

Lesson 6: When we look at nature's wisdom, we come to understand that life is a series of transitions that never end.

"Where the Soul Never Dies"

Nature, a reflection of our soul,
reveals the seasons of our lives.
Like people, earth's seasons teach us
patience, awareness, and encourage us to grow.
From the sparkle of sunlight in the doe's eye
to the sparrow elevated by the air below it's wings,
the spirit of God is this source of life that fuels our spirit
and raises us above pain and sorrow.

Only the soul can travel to this place above the clouds
where we are lifted by the breath of God.
Here, the lessons learned in nature
disclose to us that dying is a transition into life
and nothing completely disappears.
Rather, we are transformed into another realm of existence
to experience the essence of life
WHERE THE SOUL NEVER DIES.

Sam Oliver

This poem was inspired by a fellow poet nicknamed "Skeet," who I came to know through hospice. Skeet suffered for two years before her cancer reached its final stage and she was admitted into the hospice program. Skeet was a "take charge" kind of woman who loved people, fishing, gardening, animals, and especially nature.   .

She was growing weak and knew it, and on one of my visits she asked me to sit at her bedside and said, "Now, let's get down to business . . . " She wanted to tell me what she wished said at her grave. Like a good pastoral care counselor, I listened. Skeet asked me to share with others the beauty of God's creation.

Skeet told me that nature has a lot to teach people about the seasons of our lives. When we look at nature's wisdom, we come to understand that life is a series of transitions that never end.

Skeet knew that she was in the autumn of her life. She had shared with me in previous visits, dreams of people who had gone on before her to live in heaven. Her dreams gave her a sense of peace, especially when she saw visions of herself in this place of rest, free of pain. She was beginning to take an inner journey that led to a letting go of life as she knew it.

Not long after our talk, Skeet's personal winter came. I was called, along with a hospice nurse, to be present at her death. I remember the silence as we entered the room where her body lay. I felt the emptiness that comes with the loss of a friend. I remember the mixture of emotions that seemed to be swirling together like water in a drain on a street corner after a hard thunderstorm. On one level, I was glad she no longer had to suffer. On another level, I knew I would miss our time together.

Winter can create the illusion that it will last forever. Eventually, though, spring comes. After her death came a period of barrenness for me, and then one day I felt the pulse of our relationship beating again in a different way, inside my heart. I knew Skeet was more than a memory. She was a living presence. Her zest for life in the midst of dying taught me a lot about the endlessness of relationships.

Summer arrived and my relationship with Skeet fully bloomed. I knew death had not ended our bond, even though what Skeet shared with me about nature before she died had faded. A part of

Skeet will always remain within my soul. Her openness to nature and people were fresh and changing. Her outlook challenged me to grow. On days when I feel as if the sun is draining me of life, I am reminded by Skeet to pace myself, focus, and find renewal through a special gift of God's creation—the gift of the Holy Spirit.

The Holy Spirit is the fabric of our lives that connects us to one another and to nature. It enables us to live in the moment of the potential during the moment of the concrete. In other words, the Holy Spirit enables us to be a part of creating our future rather than the future creating us.

The Holy Spirit reminds us of the parallels between human beings and nature. No one knows if a seed will become a flower; a water bug will become a dragonfly; a baby will become a child, teenager, adult, or elderly, but we trust these things will come to pass. It is in our moments of hope and trust in a future beyond the physical eye that we are able to experience the Holy Spirit of life.

The Holy Spirit is something that no theologian has ever been able to fully explain. It is a state of being greater than ourselves that coexists and guides us through the transitions of our lives. It is a journey into faith, hope, and meaning greater than our present reality.

The Holy Spirit encourages us to be aware of the hidden meanings in God's creation that can guide people from this life into the next. To me, the Holy Spirit represents our internal relationships with nature, people, and God. It is the experience of being blessed, known, seen as good, wanted, and loved. It is the ability to know with assurance that life's capacities are more than just physical, emotional, and mental. It is what enables people to see potential in life that goes beyond what is seen on the surface. The Holy Spirit is an inner world that has no end and is constantly changing.

The branch blossoms, the eggshell cracks, the leaf falls, the tadpole's tail shrinks, the hibernation begins, and from the barrenness of fallow time—new life begins. In essence, nature and all of God's creation reveals that nothing completely disappears. Rather, we are transformed into another experience of life.

Nature is the soul's repose. It is ever-changing and eternal. Golden flakes of leaves baked from the summer's heat remind us of the coming breeze. The fall wind that sifts across the earth's mold cause animals to nestle in their nests and await the winter's cold. After the time of dying or "transformation" that winter brings, the air begins to warm and blossoms are born. It is the sign of new life and hope that God brings after the harshness of loss.

PERSONAL REFLECTIONS

Eternal Love

Lesson 7: Eternal love reaches into the heart and soul of an individual. It is the same love that continues to ensure the existence of the whole universe.

For a year and a half, I visited a hospice patient named Bob. We spoke many times about the joys and sorrows this life can bring. We had a lot in common. We went to the same church, both had children, and we loved our wives. Even though Bob's wife was physically dead, he spoke of her as though she had never left him. Perhaps, the difference between romantic (or earthbound love) and eternal love has to do with where one places one's attention.

Romance focuses on a passion. Usually, this passion is concentrated on a particular aspect(s) we find loveable about or in someone else. A romance centers its primary focus on some unique quality about a person who brings out the best in us through his or her presence. This is the kind of love in which we do something for another person because of what he or she brings to the relationship. Therefore, romance is a love that has been bonded as a result of something each person manifests into the daily life of another. At the same time, romance is a love united by a certain external expression(s) of who we are. When the passion is gone, so to is the romantic love.

A love that touches the soul is a relationship that reaches into the deeper dimensions and understandings of two people joined to enhance each other's life. Eternal love knows no bounds. The focus of eternal love centers its attention on what a relationship can give to another despite whether or not similar passions are shared. A relationship of this nature goes beyond something two people have in common or need from each other to bring about fulfillment. In this kind of love a fellow soul unites with a fellow soul and journeys beyond the five senses.

Even death cannot separate us from eternal love. The human mind alone cannot grasp any value in death and dying. In fact, most people spend a great deal of their time thinking of ways to avoid the inevitable. Death has become a hindrance for those who do not understand the redeeming value death can bring to us. Others have found that the death of a loved one has revealed a deeper expression of their love than the physical presence.

To deal with the notion of death in a way that brings hope beyond the physical world, we need to journey into a dimension of life where we are transformed by a renewing of our mind. This journey into the vast realm of conscious awareness, in which one is transcended into the presence of God, enables us to trace our understandings gained within this earthly life, to a reality where the body cannot travel. This is the path of the Spirit. Spirit is who we really are. It is not until we realize who we are that a trans-formation process is set in motion. From this perspective of the world and the people around us, we are able to love people and the world from a realm of reality that permeates our whole being.

I have come to believe that there are two realities in this world—love and fear. Many of us are very aware of the reality of fear. Fear has the capacity to separate us from the very source of assurance that we belong to a much greater life essence than the one we view with our physical eyes. Fear deceives us into believing that the body is all there is. No wonder great fear is experienced by many who find that their physical life is coming to a close or that a loved one they know will no longer be with them. If this is where we place the focus of our lives, it will become our reality.

Eternal love has no beginning or end, and eternal love is the only reality that truly matters. Love simply is. It is an awareness of this very moment being the only reality that reveals our essential nature. When we give our full attention to the present moment apart from living in the past or anticipations of the future, we are able to take a peek behind our accumulative thoughts and feelings to a wise old guide who has been with us all along in this life and who will lead us into the future. Even in the present moment, we are not the thoughts we dwell on or the feelings we feel. Our essential self knows we are more than a body. We are much greater than physical ideas of ourselves. The moment we accept the notion that we are more than the thoughts we think and the feelings we feel, we will have acknowledged our greatest potential for love.

Some have called these wise old guides angels. Others call this particular aspect of ourselves the Holy Spirit. It really does not matter what we call this part of ourselves. Popular religion would have us believe that we can only call this part of ourselves certain names such as: the Holy Spirit, Christ, God, etc. I am not criticizing religion, but I do challenge the use of religious labels to define the whole existence of one's understanding concerning life's essence.

If we base our highest understanding in the notions we have gained through religious beliefs, we will have made religion/belief systems our highest source of truth on the nature of the greatest source of all life, known to many as God. God, who is beyond concepts, cannot be classified. To think we can define God with a word is preposterous, and the moment we do so we will have made God in our own image and likeness. In so doing, God would be our creation, rather than the other way around. We need to trust in the very source of wisdom that created all we have known, know, or will ever know. This creator of all life is beyond our concepts.

I believe we need to listen and follow the inner director of our lives to fulfill our unique mission in this world. We need to trust, love, and accept our inner guide without judgment. We can call this inner guide whatever we wish as long as we surrender our ego or conceptual understanding and embrace our spirit. Here, we have a greater sense of self than what we have learned to this point. It is to claim our birthright. It is to realize that our greatest potential lies not in the accomplishments we make in this earthly life, but in the incarnating of our greatest sense of self (spirit) into the physical domain. From this vantage point, we are able to be caught up in the presence of the source of all life who gives us meaning and purpose in our birth, living, dying, and death. For truly, those who live their lives in the Spirit can never die. Sorrow dissipates into joy when we follow our spiritual paths, no matter where we are guided. Even our dying can be viewed as a necessary journey to find enlightenment into the greatest sense of our essential self.

It took a knot on my back to realize the things I have spoken of thus far. My doctor examined the knot and felt a biopsy was necessary. Before I received the results of the biopsy, I truly felt that my world was coming to a close. Unfortunately, I had surrounded my understandings of this world through a faith in external realities. As an ordained minister, I could tell others to trust in the spirit of God as they physically died, but I had not fully embraced this for myself.

Now, I realize that spiritual growth is a process. It doesn't matter where we are on the journey of faith, as long as we are on the journey. To me, there is a deeper part of us that knows we have an inner world within us manifesting itself into reality each moment of our lives. This spiritual part of us will never die.

Also, this spiritual part of us understands the nature of love we all share, and it doesn't really matter if we continue on in physical form or not. Eternal love reaches into the heart and soul of an individual. It is the same love that continues to ensure the existence of the whole universe.

PERSONAL REFLECTIONS

A Peace That Passes All Understanding

Lesson 8: Eternal love is so great that it is impossible to keep it to ourselves.

One day, I came in from a patient care conference at hospice. As usual, I checked my mailbox before walking to my desk. In it was a note stating that a hospice patient named Bob wanted to see me. It was unusual for Bob to request a visit, so I knew something out of the ordinary was going on.

Immediately, I phoned Bob. When he answered, I could tell he was crying. Bob wasn't one to express his emotions, so I listened intently as he tearfully asked me to visit. Although Bob said it would be OK if I came to see him at the end of the day, I knew that he could use a visit as soon as possible. Therefore, I told him that I would be right over.

My spirit moved within me as I drove to the nursing home where Bob resided. I walked into his room to find him deep in thought and filled with emotion. Bob had so much on his mind that he did not know where to begin. Slowly, the tears came. We joined hands and I could feel much warmth and intense energy radiating from him. I knew something was going on inside of Bob, as I waited for his story to unfold. He did not want to be alone as he felt these inner stirrings, and I considered it an honor to have been chosen to share this moment with him. In that moment, Bob began to share with me a wonderful journey.

As I listened to him unfold parts of himself, go deeper and deeper into his soul, I realized Bob was in a tremendous state of peace. I also learned that this spiritual peace was very disturbing to him. At that time in Bob's life, he knew that his time on earth was drawing to a close. Although Bob could spiritually celebrate being reunited with his wife in heaven, Bob was also leaving behind two loving daughters. I sympathized.

Earlier that morning, my daughter Emilee woke up from her night's sleep so sick she could hardly move. I went to work with tremendous inner pain from the fear of losing my only daughter. Perhaps this pain helped me to identify with Bob's pain. In this moment, we shared a common lot, but Bob took me even deeper than human loss, to a place of infinite peace. Our souls journeyed into the center of life where we emerged with an eternal spirit of love too awesome for one person to experience alone.

Eternal love is so great that it is impossible to keep it to ourselves. Eternal love has the capacity to reach into the deepest part of us and pull from us a knowing. This is a knowing that connects us to the source of all life, where the embracing of this knowing cannot and will not rest until our soul unites with a fellow soul in a sea of unity joined by the peace of God.

In this moment surrounded by eternity, I felt as though Bob led me to the edge of the "Great Mystery." A mystical moment that drew Bob and myself into a place where our spiritual lives could be anointed by the breath of God. In the deepest part of this union, I could feel the holy warmth of an eternal presence. We were engaged in a movement from care giving to care sharing where our souls, united by the power of peace, led Bob and I into a journey only our souls could make.

For a year and a half, Bob shared with me the love he had for his family and friends in this life. I have often wondered what kept this man alive. Bob had gone well beyond the doctors' prognosis for his life expectancy. Yet, when you got to know him, you came to know a man who had a passion for living this life in which so many people had reached into his spirit and become a part of who he was. I never sensed that death was a fear for Bob. Instead, Bob's greatest fear came on the day a family conference was called at the nursing home, a week before his phone call to me. On that day, I saw Bob's first tears. His worst fear from the past year and a half had been realized. Bob could no longer walk or be lifted without the risk of breaking a bone. A part of me was deeply saddened as I heard him say to the attending staff and his family during the conference that a man should be able to care for himself rather than be a burden to those who love him. It was in this moment of transformation that Bob seemed to begin a journey into the inner part of himself for strength beyond himself. From this point on, Bob lived in two worlds—the physical world that brought him pain and existence and the spiritual world that brought him freedom. Bob had to realize that he would always be a part of his daughters' spiritual lives before he could let go of his physical life that had become no more than a mere existence.

Before I left Bob that day, I knew his journey ahead would be difficult. Bob had spent a great deal of his past year and a half making sure that he would remain independent, so the phone call I received the following week from this very strong-willed man was a cry from the depths of his spirit.

About a month after this visit, Bob went to his eternal rest. A week before he died, he asked me to participate in his funeral. He died the day before I was to go to Hannibal, Missouri for my wife's fifteen-year high school reunion. Like Bob, I was torn between two worlds. Then, I remembered an experience from the day before Bob died that I have shared with only three people before this writing.

During a Sunday morning church service, I felt an enormous presence within me. It was very familiar, and I knew I was being filled with Bob's spiritual presence. I closed my eyes and envisioned Bob ascending into the heavens and resting on a cloud. I wondered if this was Bob's way of saying goodbye, and I returned the focus of my attention to the church service.

Although Bob died the following day, I had heard that a significant decline in his physical condition did occur that morning.

In reflection, I can't help wondering if this was my personal goodbye from Bob. Was it my personal funeral service? Did we make a connection that transcends what any ritualistic eulogy could convey? The experience felt as though we were caught up in a holy moment and articulating this inner vision does have the tendency to diminish its sacredness. I do not need these questions answered for my experience to be real, for Bob showed me in that brief encounter why he was feeling a peace that goes beyond understanding. Bob showed me that we will meet in a place where the connections we have in this world and the one to come can join. Our souls harmonize in this place led by the spirit of God who breathes into our lives possibilities beyond human understanding.

When Bob could no longer identify himself as a physical being capable of doing things for himself, he began an inner journey that went beyond earthly definitions of the self. I know that Bob was not disappointed in this inner reflection of his higher sense of self. In fact, it was quite the opposite. Bob found a source of love too enormous to experience alone. He found a peace that passes all understanding.

PERSONAL REFLECTIONS

Tears of Honor

Lesson 9: Tears are a reflection of honor.

Iris described caring for her eighty-eight-year old mother as a labor of love. Her mother had carried her for nine months, brought her into this world, and cared for her to her adulthood. Now Iris's mother was dying of cancer, and she desired to carry her mother to the threshold of eternity and release her mother into the womb of creation from which her own birth had emerged. She wanted to catch a glimpse of the power that brought her life into this world.

Iris shared with me both the good times and difficult times she and her mother had had together. During our visit, Iris and I were in the same room where her mother lay in silence. Although Iris' mother was comatose, her nurturing spirit was alive and well in the stories Iris shared. I listened as Iris weaved her mother's life into the tapestry of her own soul. She was incredibly descriptive as she told me of the joys and sorrows they had shared. I was able to draw a picture in my mind of what those events must have been like. Telling stories of her mother's life made a significant difference in how Iris expressed her grief.

The following is a list of ways we can help families and friends express their losses:

Encourage stories. Stories draw out memories and experiences that lead the storyteller beyond present thoughts and emotions. Stories lead us into our soul and allow almost forgotten memories to come alive.

In a remarkable way, our own past becomes presently alive as storytellers relive their experiences by voicing those thoughts, emotions, and experiences. These stories come to life again and awaken our spirit to the renewal of a life once lost.

Encourage faith. Faith requires us to trust in a dimension of life greater than ourselves. Faith gives us hope. Faith gives us strength. Faith gives us a reason to go on in the midst of despair.

Anyone can believe in the goodness of life while things are going smoothly. But, faith is more than believing during the good times. Faith demands our willingness and ability to trust in an overall plan for our lives beyond our own control. Sharing our faith with others reminds us to surrender our personal desires to the universal will of our Creator.

Encourage humanness. Losing someone by death causes past regrets, intentions, failures, hopes, dreams, and admirations to surface. Our memories define collectively who we are. The stories we exchange with one another make their way into our spirit and awaken us.

When we lose someone, our collective human relationships are physically severed, causing our stories to take a different shape. Pain and suffering through death breaks our heart. But, as we share our sorrow, our pain, and our emptiness, healing begins. Although we are still physically severed by death, our loved ones live on in our stories and in our memories.

Encourage ritual. Through prayer we invite God into our present physical struggles and we realize that life is more than beginnings and endings. Through prayer we are guided into an ever-present awareness beyond human understanding.

Rituals, such as anointing of the sick, communion, and funerals, serve as rites of passage for both the dying and the grieving. Here, our rituals become more than a symbol. Rituals give honor to the past and present experiences of our lives. Rituals unite us as a community of people and remind us that our lives are not on a linear timeline, but within an ever-encompassing union.

From the moment I walked into Iris's home, I suspected our visit was going to be significant. Iris had been crying when she met me at the door. Tears were streaming down her face, revealing the depth of her feelings. Her tears were more than sorrow over losing her mother. Iris said that her tears were a reflection of the honor she felt as she carried her mother back to the place where her mother brought her into this world. Here, we find that birth is not the beginning and death is not the ending, but both are a part of the unending circle of life.

PERSONAL REFLECTIONS

PART TWO:
LESSONS ON SPIRITUALITY

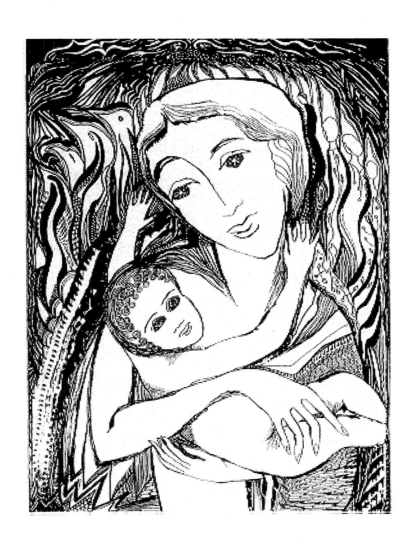

Words of God

Lesson 10: Although meaningful words are important, the words articulated in prayer aren't as vital as the depth of quality on which our awareness is centered. From eternal peace beyond the world of sound, we are able to manifest vibrations of the soul into words that incarnate God in our material world.

I pray with others often, and I sometimes take prayer for granted. I don't mean to. I just occasionally forget prayer's potential to reach into the depths of a soul the intellect can never understand. All too often, I spend much of my time in an inner dialogue talking with myself when I could be communicating with the "Divine."

Yet, communication with the Divine is blocked until our inner dialogue is silenced. In the greatest depth of our silence, a vibration emerges and whispers into existence a language only the soul can understand. This evolution from nothingness to form begins to take shape in the form of a concept. The articulations uttered from this infinite space of silence draws from eternity a kind of peace naturally felt in the act of prayer.

I pray with many patients and families almost every day of the week. Many times, I notice when I hold a patient's or families' hands, their hands begin to warm during a time of prayer. Prayer brings the calming and warming presence of God. This warmth in prayer radiates from the depth of our soul in a way that melts our external world into a solitude of silence. Prayer leads us into an awareness greater than any challenge we may face in this world. Prayer leads us into dimensions of our being that turn our greatest heartfelt sorrows into compassion. Prayer can also move us beyond our intellectual inclinations, to figure life out, to trust in a wisdom beyond our emotions and logical mind. Prayer teaches us many things, but one of the greatest lessons learned in prayer is our willingness to follow the will of God into states of awareness that we would not otherwise journey to without a deep connection with God.

Prayer is more than talking to God about our needs and wants. Prayer is an act where we acknowledge the need for continued companionship with the Creator. In order for prayer to come full circle, we have to be willing to listen for the voice of God. God speaks to us in many ways: through our family, friends, nature, illness, joy, and especially through silence.

Have you ever come to the end of a stressful day and just wanted above all else to sit in silence? In a moment of heightened calmness do you find energy from the life source known only to the soul? We all have within us, whether consciously or unconsciously, a spaciousness that draws strength from eternal dimensions and resurrects the body to go beyond its perceived potential. Prayer leads us to a presence of awareness beyond our present circumstances and leads us into mystical moments that can move us forward in faith, hope, and love.

I used to recite a memorized prayer with people. Then, I learned to pray spontaneously. Memorized prayers are very effective and I do not hesitate to say a prayer written by someone else. We have an abundance of heartfelt prayers to say to people in need written by people for special occasions, and I think they can and do need to be used when praying with people in need.

I also want to encourage spontaneous prayer. I can think of no greater feeling than being in prayer with a person and we pause and close our eyes and ask God to speak words of reconciliation through us. Spontaneous prayers move our minds and bodies into a union of unlimited possibilities. If we are conceptualizing the words coming through memorized prayer or prayers we read, we may only reach parts of ourselves we have acquired through intellectual and emotional knowledge. Spontaneous prayer has the potential to lead us into the mysterious. In spontaneous prayer, we trust God for the words needed to be spoken. Here, we have the potential to join in a cocreative process that can weave heaven and earth into a strong bond.

Not long ago, I walked by my children's bedroom. Their lights were off and my son, Luke, was asleep. In the darkness, I heard my two-and-a-half-year-old daughter repeat a meal prayer I have been teaching them to pray: "God is great, God is good, let us thank God for our food. Amen."

Standing outside my daughter's bedroom and listening to her pray sent a surge of energy through my entire body. Emilee affirmed for me the joy of prayer and the need for it. Praying is an essential part of life that acknowledges our direct connection with a continuous source of spiritual energy. Sure, I taught Emilee this prayer, and she may have been repeating this prayer because she had heard me say it many times before meals. Yet, a deeper part of me knows my daughter was engaging in spontaneous prayer, verbalizing with her best ability words that may not have made sense to her at the time.

To follow an act before we are able to conceptualize the need for prayer, to trust in the act of prayer without judging it, to pray without understanding words uttered, and to speak phrases into an infinity of silence before a critical mind calls the act of prayer into question is the kind of faith I believe God calls us to when we surrender to prayer. To model an act of faith and see my child learn to pray touches me in ways I cannot describe without diminishing the sacredness of Emilee's prayer.

What led Emilee to say these words of prayer just before she fell asleep I do not know, but I do have a hunch. I believe she was led to voice these borrowed words by her inability to articulate at her age the infinite space of silence resonating within her. Although meaningful words are important, the words articulated in prayer aren't as vital as the depth of quality on which our awareness is centered. From eternal peace beyond the world of sound, we are able to manifest vibrations of the soul into words that incarnate God in our material world.

PERSONAL REFLECTIONS

The Freeing Power of Questions

Lesson 11: Simply pondering our life's questions leads us into a dimension of ourselves where only our spirit can travel. Here, we experience freedom to incarnate into our daily lives an infinite array of choices beyond the external realities that demand our obedience.

As I sit at my computer, taking a moment to write and reflect, I am aware of just how busy my life has been over the past year. I don't often enough have the opportunity to sit and type reflective thoughts. I am married with two small children, I work full time as a pastoral care counselor at hospice, and I have friends and relatives I stay in touch with every week. On top of this, I try to weave into this a relationship with God, who gives me the opportunity to make the most of each day.

If you are anything like me, you have a difficult time focusing on what's important. We have a myriad of events to participate in, people to see, chores to do, bills to pay—all drawing our attention away from our own desires. Everyone seems to want our attention. Where can we go to find our focus? Where can we go to remember what's important? Where can we go to draw from within us our ultimate desires, concerns, and joys? Perhaps the solution to these questions do not lie in answers at all, but in the questions that draw our attention to the vast realm of possibilities hidden within the physical manifestations of life.

Simply pondering our life's questions leads us into that dimension of ourselves where only our spirit can travel. Here, we experience the freedom to incarnate into our daily lives an infinite array of choices beyond the external realities that demand our obedience. From an inner awareness, we bring to our daily lives a certain freedom—freedom from societal expectations so we may focus on our inner desires for fulfillment.

To me, religion and spirituality have served as valuable catalysts for my need to ponder the ultimate questions of my life. Is there life after death? Am I more than what I can see, feel, taste, touch, and smell? Does my spirit live in my body? Does my spirit extend beyond my body as well? These questions demand my attention and pull my awareness into the mysteries of life. I cannot articulate these mysteries without diminishing the sacred spacial quality brought forth in the mysterious. Yet, my desire to incarnate the mystical portion of who I am cannot be denied.

What are your life's questions? Do your questions challenge you to exceed your own perceived belief that life can only be lived in certain ways? If your questions do challenge you to excel, great! I have often heard that our destination is not as important as the journey. And, from my perspective, we sometimes have to lose site of where we have come, exploring new territories beyond our comfort zones, in order to end up with a broader perspective than the one with which we began. Jesus said something similar when he told his disciples, "For whoever would save his life will lose it, and whoever loses his life for my sake will find it" (Matthew 16:25). The journey of faith is nothing more and nothing less than losing sight of our own direction and following a direction beyond our own comprehension. In a sense, we have to go out of our own minds, so to speak, to begin the path of faith. When we become less interested in where we are going and more curious about who we are becoming, the journey of faith has begun.

The hospice patients I see each week demand my spiritual attention. If I focus my attention away from these inner realities, I am cutting off a fragment of who I am from what I have potential to become. We are mind, body, and spirit. To focus our attention in the area of the mind and body without manifesting the inner journey into our daily lives would be to turn our backs on the "Creator" of all beings. Yet, in reality, our lives are so busy we usually forget to pay attention to our inner journey. Thus, we end up giving more value to what we do than who we are. The truth is that both are equally important.

How can we return to the One who gives us power? How can we bring to our co-workers, families, and friends the best we have in us? How can we deal with the constant battle between our inner and outer desires? Again, I do not think we will find what we are ultimately seeking in the answers to these questions. I do, however, believe that the tensions we face have a purpose. If we become observers of these tensions, we can step back from our lives and witness a birth of awareness that sees the value of opposites coming together. In the coexistence of opposites is a spacial quality that emerges when the attraction of opposites join. This spacial quality cannot be seen, but we know it's there. It is a lot like two magnets coming together, where one is positive and one is negative. The fullness in the force engaging these two entities is beyond physical site. Yet, this invisible force is just as substantial as the forms we can see with the naked eye. In exploring our life's questions, we move beyond our physical understandings of how life appears and we connect our minds and our bodies to the Spirit that holds these tensions together.

PERSONAL REFLECTIONS

Perceptions of Reality and Death

Lesson 12: We all perceive life in our own way. Difficulty arises when we cling to a world of perception as though our own perception is the ultimate reality.

I visit many dying patients and their families each day. Often, I am amazed by how well the patients I visit appear to be accepting their approaching death. I used to think that a dying individual would be fearful, but I have found that this usually isn't the case.

A few do have a difficult time with dying. Others somehow reconcile within themselves that the inevitable is about to happen, especially if death is near. Some begin seeing their death as an escape from continued suffering. Many begin to view death as a welcomed friend.

I have seen a profound difference between dying patients who are fighting their illness to the end and dying patients who surrender themselves to a spiritual life beyond their present physical life. The difference is in their perception. Some try to hold on to a false hope that they will remain physically alive as though life in the physical domain will remain the same if "they will it so." Along with this false hope often comes anger and frustration in the dying patients' words and actions. It's like a child with a toy who is confronted by another who wants the same toy. Any interference creates anger. The anger diminishes the child's ability to comprehend and deal with reality for what it is and move on with life.

Others embrace death and accept the fact that their habitual ways of communicating to their family and friends can no longer be possible. As a dying patient and the family begin the process of accepting the death of physical connections, divine revelations emerge. Here, the dying patient becomes more than a fading memory. The dying patient becomes a medium to the spiritual for all who know the individual.

We all perceive life in our own way. Difficulty arises when we cling to a world of perception as though our own perception is the ultimate reality. Let me explain. When we perceive life to be a certain way, we try to view life from that perspective. Then, we move our lives in the direction of that perception. If this perception is in harmony with spiritual realities, we experience peace. If our perception is not in harmony with spiritual realities, our mind, body, and soul are disconnected from one another resulting in a "perceived suffering" that affects our entire being.

When we are in the perceptual world, we are in the sensual world. If we lose someone close to us, such as a family member or a friend, we suffer the loss of this relationship. Yet, we encounter many states of awareness. As we shift our attention and realize that we are human beings who have the breath of God within us, we are on our way to finding comfort in eternal experiences of life through the infinite realm of reality.

Our humanity consists of five sensory experiences or perceptions of the physical world: seeing, hearing, tasting, touching, and smelling. Each of these senses validates the human need to experience the full range of our humanity. When a loss in any of these senses comes into our life, we become sad because this particular expression of our sensual self is no longer available to us. At this point, we begin to adapt ourselves toward another way of being. Perhaps this is where trusting in the deepest part of who we are can help us. As we begin to view our life on a soulful level, we begin to experience our greatest potential in relationships beyond the physical body.

When I was a resident chaplain at a medical center in central Kentucky, I was called to a death just as I had been many times before. This death was to be my last experience at this university hospital. As I was walking to this situation, I was told that the daughter didn't know her mother had died while in the critical care unit. I was to meet her there to console her because she wanted to be with her mother when she died. I arrived in the unit before the daughter entered the room. The monitors measuring the pulse rate and the blood pressure of this woman were all on zero.

I was in the room perhaps a minute or two before the daughter entered the room and laid her head on her mother's shoulder. The nurse turned the monitors off creating a reverent silence in the room. The daughter intensely wept for a moment before she began to express her desire to be with her mother at her death. Her tears came from a depth of emotion that seemed to penetrate my entire body and soul. Words seemed insignificant, yet I wanted to say something to inspire some inclination of God's presence.

While in a state of silent prayer and before I could utter a word, the mother raised her arm and touched her daughter on the head. Needless to say, I was stunned and even more speechless than before. The nurse looked at me wide-eyed. Then, the daughter raised her head from her mother's shoulder, wiped the tears from her eyes, and stated that this was her mother's way of saying goodbye.

Was this a muscle contraction? Was it an act of God? Or, does it really matter? We all may have different ideas about what actually happened that day, and every answer would diminish the faith the daughter had in her mother's goodbye. In the conceptual world, we can find explanations for what happened. In the eyes of faith, the possibilities go beyond our perceptions. Through the eyes of faith, incredible grace becomes possible.

When our perceptual understandings of life limit our soul's longing to connect with the deepest part of who we are, we are at a crossroads. The choice is ours. Will we choose to limit our understandings of reality to just our own perceptions? Or, will we utilize the opportunity of our perceptions to validate our faith? If we choose to extend ourselves beyond the perceptual world, pathways open us to sacred journeys only our spirit can travel.

Whatever situation we find ourselves in that results in a change of a worldview, a change of a physical condition, or the loss of a loved one, how we deal with this moment of transition can make all the difference in how we move through the transformation process. As we encounter any change, our attention enters the depths of our being. Here, we begin to deal with intentions. Our intentions may be faint at first, but they are there urging us to bring order out of chaos. In our spirit, our intentions guide us forward motivated by a desire to unite the Divine with the human into a synchronized flow within our lives, manifesting physical actions.

Within our intentions, desires emerge. Our desires infuse our external lives with meaning and hope beyond our sensual world. We need to listen to the voices of our desires. At the same time, we have many voices of desire calling for our attention. Our desires will resonate something within us, reflecting clarity of thought or confusion, emotional turmoil or a stillness, the experience of caution, or the sense of something holy and sacred drawing us into the Divine. When our desires guide us to a state of peace, the next step in the transformation process is to faithfully follow this peace to its ultimate fulfillment. Our desires unfold the spiritual journey. They create new mysteries and ways of viewing the world through the inner landscape of our souls seeking incarnation. Our desires are living substances that draw our awareness into the physical world.

Once our desires surface into the world of form, the possibilities of connecting our personal experience with the lives of others are endless. No two people have the same experience. We each have our own unique human experiences. When you couple each individual experience with the Spirit of God who breathes our life into the world, we become infinite in our value. As we begin to share our own experiences with others without judging, we are able to extend our awareness beyond our limited personal understanding of life into the universal communion of soul life.

Often, we experience emotional needs in the midst of constant change, seeking our attention. As we examine our emotions, we begin to recognize that emotions are thoughts attached to physical sensations in the body, labelled with certain words to describe the feelings we have toward a particular event(s) outside ourselves. When we notice our thoughts and emotions and experience them as relatively real, transient, and in the perceptual world of form, we are free to look deeper within ourselves and to integrate a higher state of awareness into our perceptions. Emotions have the enormous capacity to sink our awareness into the inner life of our spirit, especially when feelings of loss are involved. At the same time, our emotions reveal our greatest capacity for strength when they lead us into the inner sanctuary of our soul.

Expanding to our perceptions is not easy. It requires faith in a power greater than ourselves to reveal the direction of our lives. As we surrender to this way of living, we journey beyond the conceptual world our perceptions have created and enter the world of spirit. In this sacred space, we return to a quality within ourselves that transcends perception. In the words of T. S. Eliot,

> We shall not cease from exploration
> And the end of all our exploring
> Will be to arrive where we started
> And know the place for the first time.

Four Quartets

PERSONAL REFLECTIONS

Keeping the Magic Alive

Lesson 13: Beyond our human thoughts and emotions is an awakening of the spirit from which we were incarnated into this world.

Many years ago, I believed in Santa Claus. The wonder and awe of a man I could not see was magical. This mysterious man's story lived in the heart, mind, and soul of my little world. He brought life to my inner world and made it just as real for me as the outer world. His story gave me hope. I was enchanted.

Then, one day, I was playing hide and seek with my brother and sister in the living room. While I was hiding, I discovered a present I had asked Santa to bring me for Christmas. I found it behind the organ. As I looked at this gift, my heart began to experience a myriad of intense emotions. My heart of wonder melted into a sad realization. The gift I found transformed my concept of reality, which once gave me inner joy, into a mere fairy tale.

In my work with hospice patients and families, I find a similar experience as I interact with them. Hopes, dreams, and anticipations of future experiences with their loved one facing death, sinks into the deepest parts of who they are. The physical hopes, dreams, and anticipations denied by death brings an end to a person's human story. This is why helping people to thoughtfully and emotionally close this chapter of their life is so vital. Also, I believe it is important to guide patients and families to hope, dream, and anticipate a future beyond death. Dying patients need to know that their life has brought meaning into the lives of others and that the best in them will continue on.

Many times, I am intrigued by painful emotions being expressed as a patient is dying. As these painful feelings rise, passageways open into the patient's highest self. From here, the tears that follow become a flow of divine anointings that bring about the possibility of healing. On the surface, painful emotions may seem to be all that is being manifested, but I have found more. When I listen closely, I am able to hear where these reflections of sorrow are coming from. Usually, these words of grief are coming from some dimension within the dying patient and the grieving family that mirrors an image and likeness of their spirit seeking manifestation. We all have a spirit within that cannot be seen, and it does come alive the moment our human body faces its limits.

As our emotions and thoughts are brought into the world of form, a wonderful opportunity exists. Our inner life is given a voice in the outer world. Thus, the inner self is no longer alone. Here, connections made on this level in the relationship shatter the isolation the inner self is experiencing. At this point in the relationship, we become one with those we communicate with on this new spiritual level.

Beyond our human thoughts and emotions is an awakening of the spirit from which we were incarnated into this world. Magic begins to happen as we interact with each other. Our inner self becomes aware of a connection that has, is, and will never be separated. Thus, the magic beyond the physical relationship brings a sense of wonder and hope only the soul can embrace.

Once these eternal reflections unify, we are never the same. The person who is dying resonates within our being and becomes a part of us. Then, the wonder and hope of the relationship established is assured of a continued presence that now resides in infinite love.

I am honored when I listen to the stories of people I meet through hospice. Their lives become a part of my story. Their spirit gives me hope and a reason to continue ministering to the dying. Often, I find that neither the patient nor I guide our interaction when we reach ultimate realities. As we enter the spiritual domain, our divinity manifests magical qualities of ourselves, known to our deepest sense of awareness as home.

The following are three proactive steps for families in keeping the magic of a spiritual life alive and well in the midst of grief and loss.

Be Aware of Your Insights

As dying patients deteriorate, they detach themselves from events and people that had once given meaning and purpose to their existence. A good first step is to recognize that the relationship you have with your dying loved one is beginning to take on new dimensions. Physical aspects of communicating may be coming to a close. Verbalize them. To adjust to each phase in the dying process, naming and grieving past physical rituals that can no longer be done due to physical limitations is very helpful. In each declining moment, remind yourself of what drew you to your loved one. When you do this, intrinsic values may surface. During each internal validation, you may become aware of the relationship you have with a dying loved one taking on a hopeful quality. This inward exploration may resurrect what's highest in your relationship, establishing a degree of comfort the physical losses are creating. In a sense, create an inner appreciation of the life you presently have with your loved one that may not have been known as vividly when your lives were free of your loved one's dying. Insights are inner visions or understandings of life within and beyond the physical body. Although time with your dying loved one is diminishing, your shared inner lives are eternal.

Stay Connected to Your Family and Friends

Share your personal insights with your family and friends. These insights can become helpful to others who may be experiencing difficulty in their coping. Also, these insights can bring the family together as the physical decline of your loved one reminds you how easy physical separation is. The sharing of inner dynamics the family brings to their physical connections creates a quality of intimacy needed when death touches the family. Finally, encourage others to share with you their understandings of their losses without judgment. Your stories weave your temporary human lives into the fabric of eternal life that can never be separated. Your loved one's story and how this becomes a part of your life story continues the dying person's journey.

Utilize Spiritual Resources in Your Community

Churches can be a physical reminder of the hope and faith we have in God, who unites us beyond death. Church is a place where we join one another to celebrate eternal life and the universal family of God that has no end. Spiritually, church is a place where the inner sanctuary of our souls unite with fellow souls and collectively combine our efforts guided by a higher purpose beyond our own self-interest, to live a positive life that extends peace, love, and healing for the common welfare of our community. These days, our faith communities can be a support group, an AA group, or any group in which values are guided by a higher power that connects them to eternal ways of understanding life beyond the physical.

In hospice, we place great emphasis on dying with dignity. We want our patients to die with as much physical comfort as possible. We want them to experience positive social and emotional resolutions. We want to help the dying patients and families deal with their grief of physical communications coming to a close. We want to keep the magic of their spirits alive. In so doing, we return to the mystery of life from which all emerges into this world. In the spiritual life, our souls infuse life from death. In the realm of spirit, life becomes more than a childlike fairy tale. Without the magical spirit of a childhood, all life ceases to be.

PERSONAL REFLECTIONS

Lamaze Lessons for the Soul

Lesson 14: Trust in the eternal dimension of relationships can give hope to the dying that their life will continue after their physical death has occurred.

I came to know Margot as a hospice patient. Prior to my hospice visits I had seen Margot in church, but I didn't know her. I had only been a member of the church for a short time, but she had been a member for over seventy years. Margot was elated to share the church's history and I was eager to listen. She knew its triumphs as well as its struggles. She shared with me that she felt blessed by many people in her church who had been friends. These friends were fellow followers of the Christian faith who had deepened her sense of self as a child of God. She taught me a lot about the German traditions that kept our church alive. She shared many stories about her children growing up and their family connections within the church.

Margot revealed to me her greatest experience as a church member. She learned that the universal family of God transcended her religious traditions and beliefs, especially as her faith related to her children. One day, I listened to Margot tell me how difficult it was for her to let go of her personal independence. She was used to taking care of others, not others taking care of her. On one occasion, Margot had a difficult time allowing her son to put her to bed after she had become unable to perform that function alone. Her independent nature was challenged. Margot was deeply moved to have a son care for her in this way.

About two and a half weeks before Margot died, she told me how honored she felt to be able to teach her children how to die with great faith in a loving God who she believed would transform her experience of suffering to joy. As I met and talked with her three children, Mindy, Mike, and Pat, I realized Margot had already accomplished this task.

The day before Margot died, I spoke with her son, Pat, about some of his most recent moments with his mom. He said that his mom expressed a desire to ride with the family in a limousine provided by the funeral home if the family chose to use this service. Everyone laughed when Margot's children reminded her that she would be the one in a funeral coach.

Although this moment was funny, I know Margot, in her own humorous way, was revealing something about her spirit. Margot knew her spirit would always remain in the hearts and minds of her family and friends. Soulfully, Margot did share with her family a faith in a quality of life beyond the dying body.

At the time Margot made the comment about riding in the limousine, she had begun to identify more and more with her spirit. She apparently forgot that her body would be in a funeral coach on the day of her funeral. Subtly, however, Margot reminded her family that she would be with them wherever they were from that point on. She reminded her family that their inner connections ran much deeper than physical realities. Margot taught her children how to remain united with her through "faith."

As I look back on this experience, Margot reminded me of three vital phases in the dying process: let go of independence, surrender to dependence, and live while you die.

Let Go of Independence

People need to express their grief over the loss of independence. This is a necessary part of the dying experience. Margot was used to taking care of her family and her home. In no time at all, it seemed, she had to rely on her family, her friends, and her community to care for her. This was quite an adjustment for someone who took pride in caring for herself. In a sense, it was like living a lifestyle contrary to the one she had created. For someone as independent as Margot, this adjustment did not come easy. It took time for her to surrender even a little to the role change. Whenever any of us experience a break in our routine, our balance is upset and we may feel disoriented until we accept the change and find a new balance.

Surrender to Dependence

Dying reminds us just how fragile our lives really are. When we are reminded, we have a need to share our burdens with others. We search for a direct connection with God to remind us that our spirit is not alone. We also need direct reminders from our family, our friends, and our community that we are not alone. When our inner and outer lives are supported by others, finding comfort is more attainable. When Margot could no longer climb into her own bed, she needed help from her son. Both Margot and her son expressed great humility in being part of this experience. Their experience bonded their love to a new level of understanding. As I think about their shared experience, I am reminded of the words of Christ who said, "As often as you do these things to the least of these my brethren, you have done it unto me." This was more than a son helping his mother, and a mother surrendering to this help. This was an act of obedience unto the will of God who taught us through Christ to love one another.

Live While You Die

The decision to live while dying gives purpose. When our physical faculties are in decline, we strengthen the capacity to develop inner-connections with our family and loved ones. Whether we find support from fellow church members or relatives and friends, the dying can be encouraged to live by faith and know that death cannot destroy these relationships. Trust in the eternal dimension of relationships can give hope to the dying that their life will continue after their physical death has occurred.

A few hours before Margot died, the family asked me to have a word of prayer with them. Although Margot was near death, the depth of love that she shared with her children was alive and deepening through their tears. We circled Margot's bed, held each others' hands (including Margot's), and gave thanks for Margot's living testimony of her faith through the process of dying.

To let go of independence, surrender to dependence, and live while you die are lamaze lessons for the soul. The motherly spirit of Margot did something her mind and body could no longer do. She delivered her children into the presence of God from which all life flows. Margot prepared her children for her death by giving birth to an eternal awareness of life.

PERSONAL REFLECTIONS

Creating Spiritual Awareness

Lesson 15: When a patient begins the process of detaching from a painful body that once brought pleasure, the patient searches for a way to extend awareness beyond the body.

I witness many dying hospice patients detach themselves emotionally from all of the events around them. They synchronize their thoughts to encompass a dimension of life beyond the body, i.e., imagining what heaven will be like. Then, they become vividly aware that the essence of their life is simply an awareness. Here, spiritual awareness expands beyond the mind and the body that has grounded their life.

Often, I listen to dying patients use their beliefs and imaginations to construct a view of an afterlife. Patients experience their views in different ways. Some begin this process the moment they realize their body is getting weaker and weaker. Others do this only after accepting the fact that their body will not get better. When a patient begins the process of detaching from a painful body that once brought pleasure, the patient searches for a way to extend awareness beyond the body. When this happens, the patient's mind shifts its attention from the physical body to thoughts of God.

I have observed this process many times. Each time, I am intrigued by the transformation that takes place. When I watch a patient's transformation I can't help but think of death, burial, and resurrection. The following lady is a prime example.

For the past two years, I have been visiting a woman named Victoria. She is a Catholic laywoman whose faithfulness to her church is impeccable. She prays the Rosary every day. She keeps her church, her community, and her world in her prayers. Victoria has a faith in God so deep that it encompasses every moment in her life. She is one of many hospice patients I visit who create a spiritual awareness of life beyond death.

On each of my visits, Victoria tells me stories about her life. Each of her stories reveals the way she has lived her life. Often, Victoria will share with me her curiosity about why she hasn't suffered up to this point. After we have discussed her curiosity about her personal suffering and the suffering of others, she is silent. When she is ready, we begin praying the Rosary for those who are suffering. Then, we speculate on what heaven will be like, relying on the knowledge we have both gained through the scriptures and relationships we have encountered.

During my visits, I watch Victoria's body as she talks about suffering. Her shoulders draw inward, her eyes look to the ground, and her voice weakens. After our time of sharing concerns, we are again silent. Then, we begin talking about freedom from suffering through our relationship with God. When our discussion moves away from suffering into freedom from pain, I witness Victoria's shoulders pull back, her eyes raise, and her voice strengthens with confidence in a hope greater than her present experience of life. Through Victoria I can see and experience a holy moment of transformation. First, we discuss our humanity and death. Second, we experience a burial through Victoria's silence. Finally, we encounter a renewal of our conscious awareness about life beyond the human experience.

Victoria created many events in her life: a family, a Rosary prayer group, and her own personal touch in the lives of people in her community. Her greatest creation was the love she had for God and all people. Her living testimony serves as a reminder that our devotion to God "must" come first. I don't believe I have ever visited Victoria when this message was not taught to me in some way. Although Victoria's creations will fade, her message of love will always remain. We are all creations of love. When we forget who we are, we deny ourselves joy, peace, and love.

Recently, Victoria fell and tipped over her statue of Mary. It broke. For over fifty years, she had used her statue to reflect on her faith, and she shared with me how she had acquired it. Its value certainly represents an evolution of events that connects her to her church, her community, and her universal community of faith. The statue was a reflection of her soul, which transcends the object itself. She had used the statue of Mary to experience the presence of God through continued meditation on its symbolic impressions in her life.

We have many ways to reflect on our faith. Some people use rituals, churches, the Bible, writing, nature, people, friends, family, etc., to remind them where these divine inspirations originated. These manifestations come and go in our lives, and these experiential manifestations infuse our lives with meaning. Perhaps, even the world in which we live can be used as a reminder as to "how well" we are spiritually. The way we treat each other, the way we take care of ecology, and the way we take care of all the resources available to us may be a reflection of our own spiritual journey. As we encounter our exterior life, we encounter our inner life. The world of form reveals our work, our mission, and our purpose. Sometimes we responsibly use this power within for the good of the cosmos. At other times, we use this power for our own desires. How we use it can help or hurt our world.

Life does not come from us. Life flows through us. To be creative is to join our Creator in the evolutionary process of life. The following are three ways to keep our Creator's spirit flowing through us.

Release Past Creations

The life we have created for ourselves in the past can never be retrieved except through our memory. As we retrieve this information, we can choose to detach ourselves from their results and learn from them. All of our creations belong to a source much greater than our own efforts. Our creations belong to the Creator of these opportunities. If our creations have brought joy in our lives and the lives of others, we can rejoice in them. When our creations have not brought us peace, we can boldly present them before the Creator of our lives, asking for a recreation of the event. In so doing, we may uncover a lesson that was learned, enabling us to become a better person. Thus, forgiveness is embraced the moment we do the only thing we can in these moments—release these events into the hands of our Creator who can use painful opportunities to engage spiritual growth despite us.

Remain Creative

To remain creative is to stay open to all possibilities. No one knows what life will reveal next. We need to stay open to an unlimited number of possibilities, even if they seem painful. Our Creator can artistically implant a dream, a desire, an effort for us to take hold of and create experiences unique to ourselves. As we begin to grasp the Divine's intentions for us, we understand how our dreams, desires, and efforts become our destiny.

Cocreate with God

The moment we become open to life's revelations, we can weigh the mysteries in our lives with the cumulative experiences we have had in the perceptual world. As we allow our human nature and our spiritual nature to work together, we find harmony. And, we find hope.

At the time of this writing, Victoria goes to sleep imagining what heaven will be like. The eschatological pictures in her mind comfort her. Much as an artist whose canvas cannot be drawn without an inner vision and desire to create, Victoria is cocreating with God the next step in her life. She is creating with God a spiritual awareness of life beyond her dying.

To create spiritual awareness is to realize that the life we live is not our own. Our lives are a gift from the very One who created us. As we develop our God-given talents and share them with others, we offer a sense of gratitude for the life we've been given. The love we share returns to the heart of God.

PERSONAL REFLECTIONS

Painting Pictures We Cannot See

Lesson 16: Spiritual lives cannot die. When we give spiritual connections a voice, our grieving takes on a dimension of hope. This inner hope sustains the loved ones left behind.

Tina would have been twenty-eight years old at the time of this writing, but unfortunately, she died shortly after she was born. I recently met Tina's mother in a local nursing home. She was a new hospice patient. On my first visit, I listened to Tina's mother describe her continued relationship with her daughter. Tina was to be the child that kept her mother's and father's marriage together. One day, Tina had trouble breathing. Her mother was not able to get her to the hospital in time. Tina died. Soon after her death, her mother and father divorced. Although Tina was no longer physically alive, her spirit continued to live in her mother's soul.

She was very much connected to Tina. For the first time in twenty-eight years, Tina's mother wept tears of sorrow and joy. She told me I was the first person who acknowledged her emotional pain and continued inner love for her daughter. I listened as she cried and I saw hope return. Hope lifted her face with a smile, and filled her voice with assurance, as the emotional pain in her heart poured out during our conversation. I saw her transcend beyond physical circumstances to an inner knowledge of life beyond death.

Many good people in the past tried to comfort Tina's mother by not talking about Tina. They did not realize that she not only lost her daughter, but her hope, too. Her only source of comfort all these years was her daughter's spirit. I was humbled and honored to witness Tina's rebirth as her mother gave voice to one who longed to be heard and relieved the guilt of failure Tina's mother had carried for so long.

Death cuts off physical rituals and ways of communicating that cannot be retrieved, but the spiritual conception of this mother/ daughter relationship continued to give opportunities for a sense of belonging. Spiritual lives cannot die. When we give spiritual connections a voice, our grieving takes on a dimension of hope. This inner hope sustains the loved ones left behind.

I watch many patients and their families courageously struggle with the issue of hope. "Who I am beyond physical form?" is the cry of the dying. At the same time, "Who we are beyond physical form?" is the cry of us all. I have discovered the following three ways to keep hope alive amidst dying.

Give Spirit Space

I can think of no greater damage to spirit than to judge or label its outer expression. Our spirit is so vast, it cannot be contained by physical form. When a loved one who has died returns to us in a feeling, an inner vision, or a still, small voice, we know their spirit is greater than their physical body.

When we believe our physical bodies are the only way to connect, we lose hope and allow our spiritual connections to be lost at the moment of death. Losing hope can be just as much a part of our grief as the physical loss of our loved one. We will not find comfort in grief unless we embrace our ultimate spiritual connections.

Give Spirit Physical Expression

To touch spirit is to feel tears stream down a grieving face. To hear the voice of God is to allow those tears to speak to us. Tears are physical expressions indicating the depth of our relationship that once was and continues to be. Quietly, we know that life will emerge from these tears. Tears lead our physical expressions deep within where we find comfort in our soul.

To join the human and the divine is to embrace the creator of both, to give spirit incarnation through our five senses, and to hold each moment sacred. Any manifestation into the world of form gives us a chance to externally experience another's spirit.

Witness Spirit Unfold

This is probably one of the greatest challenges all humans face. We are all fairly versed in giving care. But something wonderful happens when we allow care to flow through us. Internally, we shift from what we can do to what God can do through us. Then, and only then, will we understand what it means to be fully human and fully divine. As we recognize the obstacles that keep the spirit from working through us, we can easily remove them and discover the infinite possibilities available to us in spirit. We become open to a universal consciousness of spirit that will benefit our highest capacity for good. Every day, terminally ill patients teach me where to find our highest good. The moment a patient takes one last breath, our focus moves internally and awakens the soul.

Not long ago, I jogged near a river. I watched the wind blow the surface of the river upstream. It appeared the river was running backward. I looked again because I know the laws of physics would not coincide with this appearance. Underneath the illusion was an undercurrent moving the water down the stream as nature created it.

So it is in our lives. Sometimes the devastation of a loss can appear to take our soul in the opposite direction we would have it go. Yet, underneath all the turmoil the soul longs to connect with its loved one once again. Just as the river on my jog, what is on the surface is often deceiving. In fact, just below our grief we find our soul working constantly until it finds a connection with another soul. Here, tears melt away the veil that hides us from our soul's journey. The evolution that follows brings healing grace to our grief when our spirit unites with our deceased's spirit.

Tina's mother did not need another person to remind her that her daughter was physically dead. She had independently grieved her physical loss for twenty-eight years. Every day, she had an inner vision of what it would have been like to be a mother to Tina. Tina's mother wanted her daughter to be acknowledged as spiritually alive and well. She also needed to know that her ability to care for her daughter was not bound by physical realities. Soulfully, Tina's mother has continued to care for Tina's well-being.

Spiritual care is giving our spirit space, physical expression, and witnessing it unfold. Spiritual care nourishes our soul and expands our awareness of inner connections with people who live on after our death. Spiritual care allows us to surrender our entire being and paint pictures we cannot see.

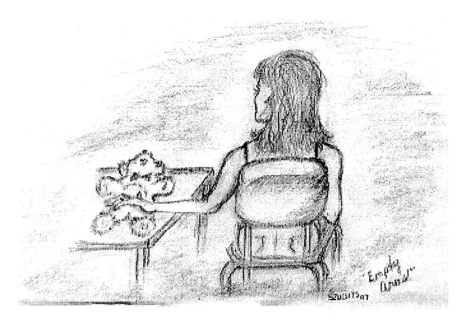

PERSONAL REFLECTIONS

Soul Retrieval

Lesson 17: As we become more aware of our thoughts and emotions (which are external expressions of our inner selves) we expand our awareness of who we really are. When we cultivate the "witness," our thoughts and emotions become teachers of eternal truths.

Recently, I met a lady who was diagnosed as having two months to live. As devastating as the news was, in a sense it awakened her spirit, and she began reviewing her life. She pondered some very painful experiences.

This lady was raised by a Catholic mother and a Baptist father. When she left home, she joined the Catholic Church, then stopped attending altogether. She considered herself nonreligious. On my first visit, she shared with me that she believed she had led a wasted life in which she had been reluctant to get close to people. She traced this detachment from relationships to a time when her cat died. The experience left her afraid to get close to another animal or person again.

These reflections have brought an understanding of the price she had paid for her emotional distance. She acknowledged low self-worth. She feared meeting God. She believed she was not loving people as God loves them. All of this was difficult for her to admit. From the death of her cat up to our meeting, she described her life as wasted.

But she knew deep down that she had not wasted her life. She was disappointed that her present life was far from what she knew it could have been. She also knew deep down where she could find peace. By her incredible experiences, this lady learned the hard way that relationships are to be valued and are vital to our lives. I felt honored that this woman chose me to listen to the story she had carried with her all these years. Telling her story brought peace within her as the spirit of love embraced her.

Although this lady went through a difficult time, she also went through a process of purification. As I listened to her share her memories, I saw a deep desire to retrieve her past and talk about how she would have lived it differently. As she talked, tears flowed down her cheeks. Her tears cleansed the pain of her losses, and those losses became small victories because she learned how to touch what is holy. I would say she learned to love as God loves.

Remarkably, this woman evolved before my eyes. I felt cleansed while I walked with her sanctifying recollections. In the same place she felt loss, she also felt her greatest hope. As she recounted her past relationships, she allowed her soul to draw strength from the past and to face the reality of her life.

Many times, hospice staff and volunteers are called on to listen to stories of regret from dying patients. Each time I listen to these stories, a piece of my own soul is retrieved and grows from the experience. So far, I have found the following three steps to a growing soul as I listen to these dying patients.

Listen to Thoughts

When I listen to hospice patients, I listen for their concepts of reality. The closer they move toward death the more their belief system changes. I have witnessed many patients shift their beliefs from what they think they have learned of the real world to an internal knowing. As they experience their inner knowledge, they set aside their concrete understandings. Their thoughts become more spacious, until they no longer need to hold their life together through concepts. In so doing, they embrace infinity.

Listen to Feelings

Feelings have a unique quality about them that thoughts do not have. Here, our attention turns to a person's ability to focus on what the body is sensing about our experiences. In their own way, feelings are impulses of information that guide us into a level of awareness that cannot be conceptualized. Feelings lead our attention to soul life. Then, our whole self rests in the acceptance that events in life are beyond our ability to completely comprehend. When the brain surrenders its limitations to the heart, the phrase "my heart goes out to you" is given expression. Here, the soul experiences a myriad of fluctuations only our spirit can bring to wholeness.

Listen to the "Witness"

Listening to the "witness" allows our relationships to be guided by a power greater than ourselves. As caregivers, we are privileged to witness the thoughts and feelings of dying patients and the family members who are left behind. As we observe the thoughts and feelings of a person's present dying experience, we witness a moment in their life where their spiritual selves may be the only part of them that can comfort their dying mind and body. Our inner awareness lies behind our thoughts and emotions. We often do not draw from our inner selves unless our minds and/or physical bodies are in danger. As we become more aware of our thoughts and emotions (which are external expressions of our inner selves), we expand our awareness of who we really are. When we cultivate the "witness," our thoughts and emotions become teachers of eternal truths.

I never know how many times I will visit a patient, but I do know that every visit I make I discover how much I lack before God and others. Yet, the instant I return my attention internally to who I am, my lack of understanding is dissipated by eternal grace. May the grace of God lead each of us to this place of equanimity. In so doing, we will find an unconditional loving presence who loves us in spite of ourselves.

PERSONAL REFLECTIONS

PART THREE:
EVALUATIVE LESSONS ON LIVING

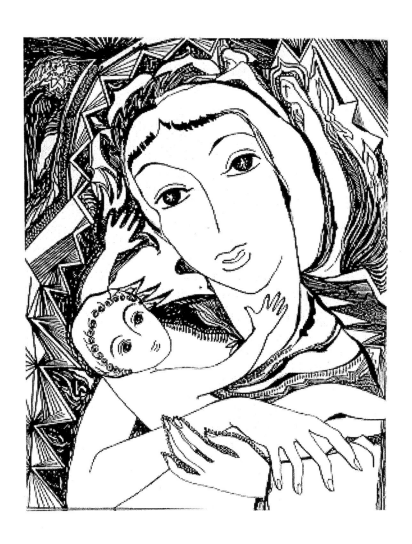

Spiritual Ethics in the Medical Setting

Lesson 18: Spiritual medical ethics gather the authority of doctors, patients, and families and place their decisions deep into the spiritual universe that governs our world.

When I was a resident chaplain at a cancer center in central Kentucky, I met a young man who was nineteen years old and had been diagnosed with leukemia. He was a Jehovah's Witness and was firmly rooted in this tradition. One day when I visited him in his hospital room, I watched videotapes with him about the Jehovah's Witness lifestyle. I learned that their commitment to spiritual teachings and family values were strong ties that created Jim's understanding of God.

For Jim to live, his type of cancer required a blood transfusion. However, Jim's faith did not allow blood transfusions. If he decided against a blood transfusion, he would die. The conflict of principles put Jim in a catch-22. His choice would decide the principles on which he would stand.

I was asked to visit Jim to help him work through his decision. The more I spoke to him, the more it became evident that he had already chosen his path. He was firm in his faith and chose not to have the transfusion. It was apparent that the staff was uncomfortable with his decision to die.

If Jim accepted a blood transfusion, his chances of living were very good. Despite the external pressures from the staff, and from giving up his future hopes and dreams, he stayed with his faith. Was Jim choosing life or death? Do we allow external circumstances to guide us? Or do we follow an eternal awareness beyond our personal understanding of life? We may all have different perspectives on these questions depending on the values that guide our lives.

Jim remains in my psyche. He has been a mentor to my faith and a spiritual guide on my path of life. His decision had not been an easy one. His own family was divided even though they, too, were Jehovah Witnesses.

This is one of many ethical issues the medical profession faces every day. Ethical ways of living our lives move us into the sacred. Here, we are talking about the guiding forces of our lives. In the past, the doctor guided much of our medical care. Now, the patient and family make decisions about medical care. Perhaps we are coming to realize that there is more to our life decisions than our own clinical, individual, and family choices. It may just be that we are returning to a wisdom that is ancient and still holds true from the first day humanity was created. That is, the choices we make influence far more than our own family and community. In fact, the spiritual implications of a person's capacity and choices have the ability to affect the entire world. Jim affected much of the hospital staff. I heard a number of conversations about Jim and everyone had their own opinion about his decision. Jim eventually died, but his faith instilled a deeper understanding of values in those of us who watched him face death with courage. He showed great strength that inspired many of us to take a soulful look at what guides our lives.

Ethical decisions draw us into our spiritual nature and call us to utilize our holiness both personally and universally. Ethics are about character. They are not defined by our present physical circumstances. Rather, ethics reveal who we are because of our external circumstances. Spiritual medical ethics gather the authority of doctors, patients, and families and place their decisions deep into the spiritual universe that governs our world. Ethics take us beyond a standard of care and move us toward universal laws of spirit.

The following are a few questions we can ask ourselves, whether we are the patient or know someone who is a patient, in discerning our medical/ethical treatment.

What Is Our/Patients' Belief System?

Our belief system can determine how we will respond to treatment options. Beliefs guide our lives. Our lives change only when we shift our beliefs. When this occurs, our mind and emotions work together to restructure the body's response to treatment. If we believe medical treatment will enhance our overall well-being without compromising our beliefs, we will most likely respond positively to treatment. If the opposite is true, we will probably undermine all medical efforts offered.

What Are Our/Patients' "Lived" Values?

Anyone can list values they would like to exhibit, but the values we exercise are the ones we live by. A thorough investigation of our "lived" values aids in building our belief systems. If our beliefs are congruent with our lived values, we will find inner peace. If our beliefs are incongruent with our lived values, we will lack potential syncronistic healing.

What Are the Influencing Forces in Our/Patients' Lives That Will Affect Our Choice of Care?

We all face influencing forces no matter what decisions we are making. Influences come from both the external and internal world. External may include family, friends, co-workers, career, church, environment, or geographic area. Internal influences may include hopes, dreams, goals, values, beliefs, self-worth, purpose, emotions, fears, etc. Sometimes our internal forces are not enough to encourage us to get well. In this case we may respond best to external medical sources that spark determination and life back into our bodies.

If We Could Choose How Our/Patients' Treatment Was Administered, How Would It Be?

Some distrust the medical profession and choose alternative healing such as homeopathic medicine. Others trust the conventional methods of treatment and have no trouble following the treatments prescribed. Our choice, again, depends on our beliefs, our "lived" values, and our environment. No matter which method of treatment we choose, as long as we are committed to that treatment, our chances for a positive outcome increase.

Where Do We/Patients Feel Our Higher Power/God Is Leading?

We can only do so much for our body. At some point in our lives our spirit will get restless and will not be content until it joins our Creator. Our body will heal if our spirit is not ready to be with our Creator. Yet, even with our best intentions, our best medical efforts, and our strongest desires to get well, we have an omnipotent dimension to our lives. At some point our soul is beckoned by God's universal will, a universal will that knows what's best for our individual lives and the collective consciousness of all humanity. It is at this point that we ultimately surrender our lives unto the very One who brought us into being.

The above questions lead us back to our beginning. They reveal life's mystical longing to go beyond our own beliefs about human life. By answering these questions we develop a deeper understanding and appreciation of the divine wisdom surrounding holistic care. When we empathetically offer care that matches the depth of spirit the patient is inviting us to, we embrace them with more than physical, mental, and emotional care. We embrace them with love.

Even though I did not agree with Jim's choice, I was able to respect his strong principles and the decision he made for himself. The ethical dilemma remains. Will our physical care and emotional support reflect the avenue in life by which the patient is being eternally guided? Or, will we take it upon ourselves to overlook the patient's ability to discern his/her own physical care? Imagine how angry and stressed we might feel if our own capable and responsible decisions were discounted by others who "thought" they knew what was best.

My deceased friend continues to remind me that there is more to life than what is visible. He taught me to look deep within myself and embrace my life-giving source. He instilled within me the importance of being true to my principles, even to the point of pain and death. He embodied, in his dying body, the presence of Eternity. He was a channel for God to speak to my spirit and enliven me with hope beyond death. As we continue to be guided by principles of ethical decision making, I trust the medical profession and caregivers will realize the intrinsic values of a patient. Only then will we honor spiritual ethics in the medical setting.

PERSONAL REFLECTIONS

Healing Relationships

*Lesson 19: Healing relationships occur inside of us
and can be inspired by relationships outside of us.*

Does faith play a vital role in the alleviation of pain in the medical setting? Does faith bring a sense of healing to people in pain? Does faith have a practical role in the health care profession? Perhaps, the answers to these questions are not as vital as our willingness to explore their possibilities. Our willingness to explore the role of faith in the alleviation of pain enhances greater possibilities for its diminishing affects. Collectively, I have heard enough stories of faith in healing arts that I want to give faith the attention it deserves. Although I believe faith does play a vital role in the care of a person in pain, individually, we determine the value we place on faith from and for our own experiences.

One of my earliest memories of healing was when I was a small boy. I remember my mother holding me gently in her arms after I fell and hurt myself. She would put bandages over my cuts and "doctor" the injury and tell me it would be OK. Of course I believed her, I had no reason to doubt that I wouldn't heal. Was my attitude toward my healing positive because I believed what my mother told me? Or, was there a part of me that simply had a blind faith in the natural healing process?

The healing process is not something tangible, nor can we examine it under a microscope. People throughout the centuries have trusted the healing process even though it remains a mystery. Since the beginning of time, we have profoundly evoked

healing through the power of faith. Whether we are aware of it or
not, faith speaks to us through our body. When we listen closely,
we know we are being directed from a very deep place within
and beyond us. It is when we listen to our body's needs that we
seek help for our pain.

We begin to seek professional advice from different types of
healers with specialties in chemical medicine, energetic medicine, herbs, and technological care to bring us comfort. We place
faith in their knowledge of the body's innate capacity to heal
itself. Professional healers call on their faith through healing
methods to counteract the body's energetic system that has
moved out of its natural rhythm of wholeness causing disease in
the body.

What brings on this mystical magic of healing? Is it the chemical drugs, technology, the doctor's word that we'll get better, or
what we believe? Or, could it be something like that of a parent's
love for a child experiencing dis-ease with a particular experience of life? Could it be that something as simple as having faith
in the power of being care for, loved, and wanted, despite the
pain we fell, alters our awareness enough to integrate a healing
response? I am suggesting that the isolating affects pain renders
may be diminished through the gift of relationships from those
willing to offer their awareness of health. The merging of "the
helper" and "the one being helped" can lead to a trusting relationship, and thus, ignite healing from a source of care beyond
our manifested forms of healing medicine.

The moment we begin to embrace someone's desire to extend
care, we begin to connect with a quality of attention the person is
willing to give. When this quality of care comes from the essence
of who we are, a sacred union develops. Both the one being cared
for and the caregiver are transcended into a holy moment guided
by the force of love. Our continued faith in that which infuses our
every breath and our relationships is united by a power greater

than ourselves. In this moment, a healing faith emerges from a willingness to trust that our pain will lead us to healing.

Healing relationships occur inside of us and can be inspired by relationships outside of us. The following is a list of nine healing relationships we encounter in healthcare.

Our Relationship to Pain

Pain is a hurtful sensation that comes from within us and outside us. When we first experience pain, we immediately form a relationship with it. As we experience the different aspects of pain (physical, mental, and emotional) we can begin to make it a part of us or we can deny it. Most often, we have the tendency to keep the pain at a distance and try to continue our activities in spite of the pain. Instead, perhaps we can learn to utilize pain as a messenger for healing exploration.

When we try to keep pain separate from us, we only create further disease. The moment we realize we cannot escape the reality of our pain, the opportunity for self-discovery elicits an opening for healing. In a sense, establishing a relationship with our pain heightens our awareness of its different qualities. Here, we have the ability to be guided by our pain. We can give pain our "gentle" attention, allowing the pain to shape and possibly even change its qualities. The moment we shift from getting angry about stubbing our toe, to begin observing and caring for it, our pain messages change. We may not be completely free of pain, but our pain does make a shift in our conscious awareness of it.

Our Relationship to Desire

Desire is empowering. Desire is transformational energy drawing us to a coveted states. Desire is trans-form (beyond one's present state of awareness). It utilizes the formless states of awareness and creates a shift in our attention from what we fear to that for which we hope. Shifting our attention may be just enough to loosen the grip of our all-encompassing burden of pain. Once our desire unites with our present state of pain, faith in a higher power/God, awareness of a healer, or simply a desire for pain relief opens unlimited opportunities from the formless states of our being.

In this state of awareness, the incarnation of spiritual healing is rooted in faith. This faith creates a connection to the universal love governing our universe. At this point, the results of connecting to a higher source of power greater than ourselves can bring a sense of comfort. We may experience a sense of comfort, or we will be given the gift of endurance. In either case, we are offered the gift of grace. When we look closely at these gifts, we know we are not alone in our pain.

Our Relationship to Comfort

Comfort is a natural state of awareness. It is like a soft, warm blanket to the mind and body. We know this state because of the peace we feel when that warm blanket is wrapped around us and life is in flow. Perhaps, our memory/experience of this state alerts us when life is no longer in flow with the natural state of comfort. Comfort is also like an anchor. It is strong and stable. For many of us, it is an ideal state of awareness we hope to attain. Our ideal state of comfort can give us hope in the midst of despair. This hope can encourage us to continue seeking that which we desire, usually an active healthy life.

The awareness of our comfort state can give us an idea about how far we need to journey when we want to draw near to our idea of comfort. Our awareness of our comfort state can be a guiding light through the dark areas of the soul where pain can often lead us. Sometimes, our awareness of comfort gives us the encouragement we need to move our awareness out of the darkness and into a desired state of grace. Therefore, the journey toward comfort is our own conscious decision to embrace pain's hopefulness by letting go of its disadvantages. When we step into the gap between embracing comfort and letting go of pain, our pathway into the spirit is opened. We are then guided by an unseen higher force of life, much greater than our pain.

Our Relationship to Expectation

Expectations, much like beliefs, are anticipations of what is to come. Often, it is hard enough to deal with our own expectations regarding pain. But when we react to others' expectations on how our pain should be, our thoughts concerning our pain get distorted, and this can sometimes increase our pain experience. In other words, we listen to our pain differently when we embrace others' opinions concerning it.

Therefore, understanding our relationship with our expectations can teach us to be open to our deepest sense of self, revealing the reality of our situation. This does not mean that we do not ever integrate what others share with us. Instead, a discerning approach to all information we receive through our senses allows us to integrate all resources available (e.g., community, family, friends, ourselves, church, health care professionals, and the God of one's understanding).

After becoming informed to some degree, we are ready to explore our expectations. This is a process of trial and error until we find the right combination that will lead us to a state of grace. Thus, self-imposed limitations are left behind and we begin to surrender our lives into the infinite. Often, what we believe to be possible becomes our reality.

Our Relationship to Intention

Expectations give authority to intentions. Intentions are firmly fixed states of awareness where one focuses on a specific outcome. Intentions unite the unmanifest with the manifest, creating actions either of harmony or lacking harmony.

When harmony is generated, we become more aware of our body and our environment. Harmony creates peace, and a natural flow of energy is stimulated bringing new life to the one seeking healing medicine not made with human hands. When we are clear on our intentions, subtle energy incarnates sensory responses that were not there before the act of an intention.

Our Relationship to Surrender

Surrender is the act of giving our personal power over to someone or something. As we surrender our pain, our desires, our comfort, our expectations, our intentions, our attitudes toward medicine, and our feelings into a power greater than ourselves, we begin a spiritual walk. Here, our soul speaks to us from an infinity of silence. Our soul beckons us to embrace all qualities of our being by beginning the process of merging with spirit.

We may not find complete physical healing in our journey of the Spirit. However, the greater healing comes in our willingness to surrender into a healing relationship with our Creator, despite what happens to us physically. As we surrender our whole self into our Creator, we have surrendered into unconditional love. This is the ultimate form of trust and the deepest kind of love.

Our Relationship to Medicine

Our attitudes, beliefs, hopes, and anticipations will to some degree determine how we will respond to the type of medicine we choose to enter our energetic system. More than digesting a pill, accepting chemotherapy, or utilizing technological care, we are internalizing an entire method of healing. If the choice of treatment is made for us and if it is against our personal health care preference, chances are our bodies may not respond to treatment.

Therefore, it is very important that good communication between the caregiver and the patient be established so the type of treatment chosen is best for the patient. On the other hand, there may be cases in which the patient needs to have decisions made for him/her due to lack of mental/emotional capacity to make viable decisions. Here, a trusting relationship is important between the caregiver, the patient, and the patient's family.

Our Relationship to Feelings

A vital element in healing relationships is feelings. When we love another entity, we feel warmth toward it, be it a person, place, or thing. Feelings of the heart give us the potential to open or close our deepest longings. They function as a barometer and tell us when life is safe or unsafe. In cooperation with the mind, feelings also help us regulate the intensities of our passions.

Feelings help us connect with each other in a way that would not otherwise be possible. For example, we can empathize the loss of another's spouse in death because we can feel lost hopes, dreams, future anticipations, and collective experiences similar to those that held the relationship together. We can share in the joy of new parents and renew birth within ourselves. Feelings remind us we are alive. They remind us when we have energy and when we lack vitality.

Our Relationship with the Soul/Spirit

As we experience a relationship with the Spirit, the fullness in the formless offers new energy to our human relationships. Often, we seem to be drawn to the energy people radiate rather than to their personalities. When our energies meet, humanity and divinity intersect. The energy generated from our human relationships has the potential to either empower, balance, or lower our energy level.

When we hear someone play the piano, we resonate with the music. As long as someone is playing on key, we feel the harmony. When a wrong note is played, it creates a disturbance in our minds and bodies. Pain is similar to this illustration. It signals disharmony, or the inability to synchronize the myriad of vibrations that inhabit our body. Symbolically, the piano represents our body, the piano player represents our mind, and the music represents the energy/vibrations we experience in our beings. Inside, we have the knowledge and ability to tune any part that is off key and find our way to harmony. It is the same part of us that breathes life into our bodies. It is the relationship we have to that which infuses our lives with an awareness of a life beyond our pain. It is our relationship with the Spirit.

*   *   *

As a counselor for hospice, I am privileged to witness many relationships from the formless states of our being. You can see how these nine healing relationships parallel the human experience. Each of these qualities of attention can be used for self-reflection or they can be used in the care of patients, families, and friends we meet. These healing relationships (see Figure 1) rely on our ability to sense/feel the force of love that pervades us, guides us, and leads us home. Home is that place of harmony where we can let ourselves be who we are. It is a place of peace. The feeling of being at home is a state of awareness that will lead our spirit into our highest state of gratitude. It is here that our journey ends where it began.

The deeper our faith is created in the Holy, the larger the shift in our awareness of those for whom we care. At the same time, those we care for can raise our awareness of the Sacred. Many times, someone else's pain has the potential to reflect the personal pains we have grown through or have yet to discover. Herein lies the mutual need of the patient and the caregiver to rely on a higher intelligence to guide relationships. As a collected body, where two or more people or states of awareness are gathered, we find the guidance of our Creator. Here, our Creator calls us to a higher wisdom. In this awareness, we can come to realize that the love shared does not come from us. Rather, the love shared comes through us. In this quality of attention, healing relationships are joined on a sacred journey.

FIGURE 1. Healing Relationships Diagram

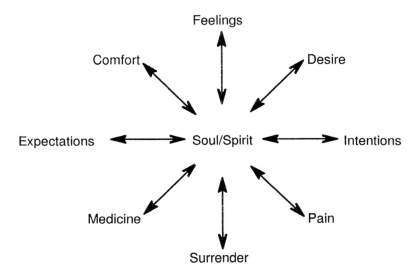

Note: Each of these interconnected relationships have different qualities and intensities. They are not levels of relationships, rather, they reflect how we are interdependently bonded to the Soul/Spirit.

PERSONAL REFLECTIONS

Facing the Unknown:
A Structured Experience

This structured experience is specifically designed for anyone seeking a clearer vision about the unfamiliar experiences in life. Its purpose is to help caregivers, family members, and medical/ support staff experience what an individual may face in the "unknown" journey toward death. This exercise goes beyond helping someone who is dying. It gives insight to anyone who might face unfamiliar experiences such as: tragedies, divorce, major illness, marriage, children, and death.

Procedure

1. Divide the group into pairs. Have one person be led around the room blindfolded by his/her partner.
2. After about five to ten minutes of being blindfolded, have the partners trade places.
3. Then, reunite the group and discuss the experience.

Discussion

1. What was it like to lead someone blindfolded? How did you feel knowing you were responsible for another's well-being?
2. What was it like to be blindfolded and led by someone else? How did you feel when you were being guided in darkness?
3. Did your reactions throughout this exercise relate to the way you move through transformations in your life? In what ways?
4. What part of the exercise made you feel more comfortable— leading or being led? Were you able to trust your leader as

well as you expected your leader to trust you when you were leading?

5. In what ways do you think this exercise relates to life experiences you cannot foresee (e.g., sickness, job change, divorce, death)? How much or how little do you think you allow your Higher Power/God to lead you through these experiences?

6. What have you learned about trusting in others and God in situations when you need help?

PERSONAL REFLECTIONS

Reflections

What the Dying Teach Us is a book about living. These stories are about living each moment of our lives filled with love, hope, and gratitude. Dying people teach us to live as if each moment is a gift. When we live with the intensity that each moment is precious, we accumulate a lifetime of wisdom and wealth consciousness that can only increase with the passing of time. Let me repeat this. When we live as though each moment is precious, we accumulate a lifetime of wisdom and wealth consciousness that can only increase with the passing of time.

I owe an abundance of my wisdom and wealth consciousness to the dying people I have been privileged to serve. The dying have taught me the meaning of life's most precious commodity—love. I have sat at the bedside of a dying person. I have sat with family members at the bedside of their dying loved one. I have witnessed invisible bonds created and souls forever linked. Dying people have the capacity to guide their families and friends from chaotic thoughts and emotions to spiritual freedom. Dying people remind us that eternity awaits us all. Most of all, dying people teach us that the lessons we learn about living come from the essence of who we are. I would like to end where we began—poetically.

"Our Relationships Are . . ."

Gentle droppings,
like rain from heaven,
sending silent vibrations
that fall to the ground

and then speak to us
the moment they touch the earth.

These unique expressions of wonder
that draw our awareness
into an ever encompassing union
between silence and sound
swirling in our midst
are the sounds of God.

The vibrations are births and deaths
of infinite possibilities
and dance through our souls
like endless streams
in the eddies of time
that cannot be measured.

Sam Oliver

PERSONAL REFLECTIONS

Bibliography

Eliot, T. S. *Four Quartets.* 1943. New York: Harcourt, Brace, and Company.

The Oxford Annotated Bible. 1962. New York: Oxford University Press, Inc.

Index

Page numbers followed by the letter "i" indicate illustrations.

Order Your Own Copy of
This Important Book for Your Personal Library!

WHAT THE DYING TEACH US
Lessons on Living

_____ in hardbound at $29.95 (ISBN: 0-7890-0475-5)

_____ in softbound at $14.95 (ISBN: 0-7890-0476-3)

COST OF BOOKS_____	☐ **BILL ME LATER:** ($5 service charge will be added)
	(Bill-me option is good on US/Canada/Mexico orders only;
OUTSIDE USA/CANADA/	not good to jobbers, wholesalers, or subscription agencies.)
MEXICO: ADD 20%_____	
	☐ Check here if billing address is different from
POSTAGE & HANDLING_____	shipping address and attach purchase order and
(US: $3.00 for first book & $1.25	billing address information.
for each additional book)	
Outside US: $4.75 for first book	
& $1.75 for each additional book)	Signature_____
SUBTOTAL_____	☐ **PAYMENT ENCLOSED: $**_____
IN CANADA: ADD 7% GST_____	☐ **PLEASE CHARGE TO MY CREDIT CARD.**
STATE TAX_____	☐ Visa ☐ MasterCard ☐ AmEx ☐ Discover
(NY, OH & MN residents, please	☐ Diner's Club
add appropriate local sales tax)	
	Account #_____
FINAL TOTAL_____	
(If paying in Canadian funds,	Exp. Date_____
convert using the current	
exchange rate. UNESCO	Signature_____
coupons welcome.)	

Prices in US dollars and subject to change without notice.

NAME _____

INSTITUTION _____

ADDRESS _____

CITY _____

STATE/ZIP _____

COUNTRY _____ COUNTY (NY residents only) _____

TEL _____ FAX _____

E-MAIL_____

May we use your e-mail address for confirmations and other types of information? ☐ Yes   ☐ No

Order From Your Local Bookstore or Directly From
The Haworth Press, Inc.
10 Alice Street, Binghamton, New York 13904-1580 • USA
TELEPHONE: 1-800-HAWORTH (1-800-429-6784) / Outside US/Canada: (607) 722-5857
FAX: 1-800-895-0582 / Outside US/Canada: (607) 772-6362
E-mail: getinfo@haworth.com
PLEASE PHOTOCOPY THIS FORM FOR YOUR PERSONAL USE.

BOF96